# HANDLING YOUR HORMONES

## The "Straight Scoop" on Love and Sexuality

### Jim Burns

**MERIT BOOKS**

A Division of Merit Media International
Laguna Hills, California

Scripture marked NIV taken from the *Holy Bible: New International Version*. Copyright © 1978 by the International Bible Society. Used by permission of Zondervan Bible Publishers.

Scripture marked RSV taken from the *Revised Standard Version* of the Bible. Copyright 1946, 1952 © 1971, 1973. Used by permission of the National Council of Churches.

Scripture marked LB taken from *The Living Bible*, copyright © 1971, Tyndale House Publishers, Wheaton, Illinois 60187.

Selection from *Sex, Love, Or Infatuation: How Can I Really Know?* by Ray Short copyright © 1978 reprinted by permission of Augsburg Publishing House.

Selection from *The Stork Is Dead* by Charlie Shedd, copyright © 1968; used by permission of Word Books, Publisher, Waco, Texas 76796.

Selection from *The Private Life of the American Teenager* by Jane Norman and Myron Harris, PhD. Copyright © 1981 Jane Norman and Myron Harris, PhD. Reprinted with the permission of Rawson Wade Publishers.

Handling Your Hormones: The "Straight Scoop" on Love and Sexuality
Copyright © 1984 by Merit Books
A Division of Merit Media International
Laguna Hills, California 92653

Library of Congress Catalog Number: 84-60033
ISBN 0-915929-01-5

Printed in the United States of America.

To
Doug Webster and Doug Fields,
friends and co-workers
who by your zeal for life and ministry
challenge me to keep my priorities straight.


Special thanks to
Cathy
for your constant support
and ministry of "lending" me to others.

Donna Gibson
for your affirmation,
your positive attitude, and your typing.

Wayne Rice
for planting the seed
to write on a subject desperately needed
by youth workers in youth ministry and education.

# Table of Contents

# Preface

I've decided that students deserve the "straight scoop" when it comes to discussing sexuality. During my last ten years of working with students, I've had the privilege of talking with them about their sexuality and they've taught me a lot. They've taught me, for instance, that they are mature enough to handle discussing even the most sensitive issues. They have been willing to be open, honest, and often quite blunt when they ask questions or offer their opinions. They have also trusted me with accounts of their own experiences and of lessons they learned the hard way. (Since we all can learn from these real-life situations, I've changed my young friends' names and included their stories here.)

Overall, I sense that students today truly desire to be all that God wants them to be. I've met hundreds of Christian and non-Christian young people who are genuinely interested in hearing a Christian perspective on the issues they face every day. I'm afraid, though, that too many students have an incredibly warped idea of God's view of sexuality. I find myself telling them that God is not the great kill-joy when it comes to sex. He created sex, He sees it as very good, and because He loves you He wants the very best for you.

An outgrowth of this dialogue with hundreds of students is this book. *Handling Your Hormones* is made up of twenty-one chapters. I've tried to make the chapters easy to read, short, and to the point without, I hope, sacrificing too many important details. At the end of each chapter, I've placed questions which can serve as discussion starters for youth ministry education or family discussion time.

In addition, there is a *Handling Your Hormones* growth guide available for use in conjunction with this book. It may be used by an individual working alone or by a group of students working with a leader. It will guide young people into further thought about and discussion of the issues raised here.

I apologize if I offend some people for being straightforward in my discussion of sensitive issues. I know that even within the Christian community there is much diversity of opinion regarding sexuality and the issues I raise here. I know some people will not feel comfortable with my leaving some of these issues open-ended. Writing from my own Christian perspective, I have tried to put together a book that touches all the issues and encourages readers to deal with their sexuality in both a healthy and a godly manner.

Jim Burns
Newport Beach, California

CHAPTER 1

# The Story of Tony and Linda

When I first met Linda, I knew that she would be a real asset to our youth group. She was enthusiastic and fun-loving, and when it came to talking seriously about our faith in Christ she could settle down and really dig in to the Scriptures. What a joy to be around! Now, two and a half years later, Linda sat in my office and sobbed uncontrollably. Her story went something like this . . . .

Although she had dated in high school, she had never really been serious with anyone until Tony came along. Tony was in the leadership core at church. He was popular at school, active in student government, and a real gentleman. At first, most of their dates were double dates or church functions. Very quickly they both fell "head over heels" for each other. For Linda, life began to revolve around Tony and the time they spent together.

A few weeks passed into a few months and the "perfect couple" began to spend more and more time together. After youth group instead of going to the hamburger stand with the rest of the gang, they would make an excuse and end up spending an hour or so kissing. They both had high moral standards, but they were so much in love that over the next few months they found themselves slipping, in Linda's words, "from light kissing to heavy kissing to light petting to very heavy pet-

ting." Slowly but surely their dates had changed from
doing fun and active things to situations in which they
"could be close." Almost every date was filled with "very
heavy petting."

Sometimes Tony and Linda would talk about their
relationship. Although they were both in high school
and wanted to go to college, marriage was a possibility.
Now, however, both Linda and Tony felt guilty about
their physical relationship. They tried to talk about it but
it was a difficult subject to discuss. Although they both
tried to "stop being so physical," it was getting harder
and harder to stop. They found themselves communicating less and less verbally and more and more sexually.

The Linda who now sat in my office was a serious
young woman struggling with guilt and confusion. It
was difficult for her to share her experiences. She and
Tony had been, in Linda's words, "going all the way" for
about two months. The night before, though, Tony had
opened up to her and shared his true inner feelings. He
loved her, but he felt tremendous guilt about their physical relationship, school was going badly, and he wanted
to be more involved with church. Although he loved
Linda, he felt that the best thing to do was to break up.

Linda was crushed, yet she knew that most of what
Tony was saying was true. She came to my office looking for answers. She still wanted to be with Tony and she
desperately wanted to know how to overcome sexual
temptation. Linda had found in her Bible a verse that
she believed to be true, but she didn't quite know how to
apply it. It says: "No temptation has overtaken you that is
not common to man. God is faithful, and he will not let
you be tempted beyond your strength, but with the
temptation will also provide the way of escape, that you
may be able to endure it" (1 Cor. 10:13 RSV).

Linda believed that God is faithful and she recognized that her temptation was common to others. Her problem was trying to figure out a way to escape her temptation and remain true to her convictions. We continued to talk for some time and came up with . . .

## SIX POSITIVE GUIDELINES FOR OVERCOMING SEXUAL TEMPTATION

### Talk About the Problem with Your Girlfriend or Boyfriend

If you don't feel comfortable talking to your boyfriend or girlfriend about your physical relationship, yet you continue to go farther than you think is right, then you have a problem. A good relationship includes open communication; in a good relationship the guy and girl should be willing and able to talk about the problem. When Linda finally did talk with Tony, she found out that he had the same guilt feelings that she did. By the way, talk about your problems over a soft drink or while walking home from school, not right after you've slipped.

### Set Standards

The best advice our premarital counselor gave my wife, Cathy, and me was to set standards *before* becoming swept up in the heat of emotions. Set standards that are right for both individuals involved. Again, over a soft drink, talk about your physical relationship and decide what your limits will be. Then if temptation comes your way, it will be easier not to violate your conscious decisions.

## Plan Dates That Will Be Fun and Enjoyable

When Joseph was tempted to lie with Potiphar's wife, he ran out of the house to flee temptation. He didn't even take time to pick up his coat! (See Gen. 39:2-15.) One of the best ways to avoid sexual temptation is to stay away from places where it is easy to be tempted. Plan dates that are fun and enjoyable. Double dates, for instance, can often be more fun than "single" dates. Also, in a recent poll of high school students, an overwhelming 92 percent said they would rather go on a "creative cheap date" than on an "expensive romantic date." Plan your dates in advance and keep away from "parking" spots and dark roads!

## Pray Together

As a Christian you will, I hope, desire to be going out with other Christians. A great way to grow in your faith and develop a better relationship with your boyfriend or girlfriend is to pray together. Praying together draws you closer to God and to each other. Praying together helps you set proper priorities for your relationship. And, naturally, praying together as a couple will help both of you resist sexual temptation.

## Break Up

One of the hardest things to do is to break off a relationship. We have often become dependent on our dating partner and wonder if anyone else will ever go out with us. There is no easy way to break off a relationship, especially one in which you have been sexually active. Yet many times the very best thing for both of you would be to break up. If your relationship was "meant to be," you can always get back together later on when you've both become more mature.

### Allow God to Be a Part of Your Dating Relationship

People of all ages can really struggle to allow God to take an active part in certain areas of their lives. This is certainly true when it comes to sexuality. For some reason it is difficult to give God this area of life. I think sometimes we're afraid God will be a kill-joy.

If it's true (and I think it is) that God cares about every area of our lives, then He definitely cares about our sexuality and wants the best for us. If you, as a Christian, allow God to take an active role in your dating life, you'll find it easier to flee temptation.

### Epilogue

Tony and Linda decided to break up. (It wasn't easy!) A year and a half later both are doing much better. Tony has gone away to college, has gotten involved in a Christian club on campus, and now says that he has really pulled his head together. He also says that he has been dating a Christian girl who's helping him live up to his Christian standards in his dating life. Linda worked full-time after high school and went to a community college at night. Next year she'll attend a Christian college. She says that she has learned to work through a lot of hard times, and she quotes James 4:8 (RSV)—"Draw near to God and he will draw near to you." She hasn't dated much in the last year and a half, but is looking forward to some positive experiences at college.

**Things to Think About**

• Have you known people who were in a situation similar to Tony and Linda's? How did it work out?

• What do you think Paul means in 1 Corinthians 10:13 when he talks about sexual temptation?

• How do you feel about the suggestion to pray together to help overcome temptation?

• What do you think it means to allow God to become a part of a dating relationship? What are some practical ways in which a couple can include the Lord in their times together?

# CHAPTER 2

# How Far is Too Far?

I wish I had a dollar for every time I've been asked "How far is too far?" or "Are we allowed to pet?" or "What does the Bible say about petting?" I'd be a rich man! This is, of course, one of the big issues we must face when dealing with our sexuality. Sometimes I wish the Bible were more explicit when it comes to this subject. But it's not. (Believe me, as a teenager I thumbed through the pages of the Bible looking for answers myself!)

The problem lies, I think, in the fact that most people ask the wrong questions. We shouldn't ask "How far *can* I go?" Instead the question is, "How far *should* I go?" The issue is not "Am I allowed to pet?" but rather "Should I pet?" People today are often looking for black and white answers. When it comes to the subject of petting, however, answers aren't easy and there definitely is a gray area.

First, let's define petting. Petting is touching, caressing, or fondling intimate parts of another person's body. There is no manual that says French kissing is okay but fondling the breasts is not okay. In fact, there is no manual to even say what petting is and what it is not. So for the time being, let's keep it as simple as the definition in this paragraph.

Perhaps a more important question than "What is

petting?" is "Why pet?" This is where we might get some real insight. In his book *How Far Can I Go?*, Larry Richards says, "Biologically, petting isn't designed to *satisfy* our emotions, but to *stimulate* and *excite* us, and lead to the fullest expression of sex in marriage" (my italics).[1]

He's right. Petting and arousal (arousal means experiencing sexual excitement) at times can be synonymous. Petting leads toward the ultimate sexual satisfaction—intercourse. Now don't get me wrong. I don't believe that every couple who is into petting will have intercourse. It is important, however, to understand that petting is not designed to satisfy our emotions or our physical desires. Instead, petting is designed to stimulate and excite those emotions and desires.

Something else to think about is that too many times petting is focused simply on personal pleasure and not on the other person. Some people in a heavy petting relationship lose sight of their special friend as they try to stimulate and satisfy their own sexual desire. Petting can become a self-centered experience rather than an effort to communicate love for another person.

The other thing that is important to mention about petting is the scientific fact that petting is like some drugs: it often takes more and more to satisfy. I've spent time with too many couples who have started their physical relationships innocently, but because of the strong drive toward sexual fulfillment in intercourse they have found themselves guilt-ridden, pregnant, or facing a broken relationship. Young people must realize that within every normal human being there is a built-in sex drive. We thank God for it, yet we also must control it. And with God's help we can control it. Who we place in the driver's seat can make all the difference when it comes to our sexual experience.

Because our sexuality is so important to us, we need

to count the cost before we become physically intimate. I think about Janet as I write that sentence. Janet was a lonely girl in my youth group. She started dating one of the popular guys at her school, and, in her words, "fell madly and passionately in love with him." After they broke up, she slipped into my office one day sobbing: "I feel mad. I feel cheap . . . . I have high standards and now I don't even like him! . . . How could I have given so much of my body to someone I thought I liked but now can't stand? . . . I sure didn't count the cost!"

That's real insight for a sixteen-year-old. Unfortunately Janet learned the hard way and after the fact that her sexuality was personal and that if she gave herself freely before marriage she would probably regret it later. I hope that others will not have to go through the pain that Janet experienced in order to learn what she learned.

In this chapter, I've tried not to use scare tactics. All I want to do is give you some facts to think about. Petting is serious business. I'm not writing for the promiscuous teenager, though; I'm writing for the person who is curious about sexuality and yet wants to be all that God wants him or her to be. Having discussed some of the problem areas, now let's look at some of the answers.

Unfortunately, there are no easy answers. Most of the Christian books on youth and sexuality simply say, "Don't pet until marriage." I understand the reason those writers say this. If people followed this advice, they would save themselves from a lot of heartache and sorrow. Consider for a moment that the average person falls in love three to five times before marriage.[2] If heavy petting is part of each relationship, there will surely be some confusion as well as pain and guilt when it comes to sexuality.

My answer is not as simple as "don't do it." The odds are that you will have a petting experience before marriage. What I want to do, however, is to save you as much grief and confusion as possible. As I said earlier, the Bible is silent on the subject of petting. Throughout the Scriptures, though, we see clearly God's desire that sexual intercourse be saved for your marriage partner. But what about all the other actions from kissing to fondling sexual organs?

I think an important question to ask is "What would be pleasing to God in our relationship?" When we begin to view our relationships with this question in mind, we begin to look at our sexuality from a positive perspective rather than a negative one.

For ten years I've given students an exercise in setting standards for themselves. (The exercise is in the *Handling Your Hormones* growth guide, a companion to this book.) I'm always amazed at the maturity I see as we consider the question "How far should I go?" It is important to think about this issue and to set standards for a physical relationship even before a relationship develops. Never try to set standards in the midst of passion. Instead, thoughtfully establish the standards for your physical relationship that you feel would best glorify God. (Remember that your body is the temple of the Holy Spirit. [1 Cor. 6:19]) Think, too, about what would be best for your relationship with your boyfriend or girlfriend. I think you'll agree in the long run that what is best for God will definitely be best for you.

---

### Things to Think About

• In your own words, how would you define "petting"?

• Why do people have such a difficult time setting

standards for their sexual behavior?

• Do you think guys or girls are more interested in petting? Or do you think both have about the same interest?

• For a practical exercise in establishing standards for yourself, refer to the *Handling Your Hormones* growth guide. Complete the chart entitled "How Far Should I Go?" with a group or alone. Decide where you would place each experience listed.

# CHAPTER 3

# Why Wait?

Tracy and Ron made an appointment to see me in my office. Although I barely knew them, I did know that they had been going together for some time. They walked into my office, sat down, and got right to the point. Ron started the conversation by saying, "Last week Tracy and I made love for the first time. It brought us even closer together. We love each other a lot. We're planning to get married in a few years and we want to know why we should wait until we're married to have intercourse!"

I asked Tracy what she thought. I think she was a little stunned that Ron had opened up so quickly, but she nodded her head to indicate that she had the same question. Tracy also had a few more reservations about premarital intercourse than Ron did. She explained, "I did feel really close to Ron, but I've been dealing with a lot of guilt since then. And I'm afraid I might get pregnant or something!"

I really liked Ron and Tracy. I appreciated their openness and their desire to make the right decision. We talked for two hours, and during those two hours they shared more of their dreams and doubts. Yes, they did love each other, but both felt that they were too young to seriously consider marriage. It also came out in the conversation that Ron was much more interested in having sexual intercourse than Tracy was.

When they left the office, I felt that I'd made two new friends. They wanted to see me again, but both of them would be away from our town for a total of six weeks for various reasons. Tracy asked if I would think about why they should wait, write them a letter listing the reasons, and then send copies to both of them to think about and discuss together when they returned. That was a unique request, but I said I would try. We exchanged addresses, hugged each other, and said good-bye for six weeks. Here's the letter I wrote them:


Dear Ron and Tracy:

You are two very special people. I think God has great things in store for both of you. I appreciate your willingness to be all that God desires you to be. Our time together on Friday has really made me do some heavy thinking and even some extra reading on what you called "the big dilemma."

Let me preface what I'm going to say by reminding you of what I said on Friday. I realize that many well-meaning people make the mistake of "going all the way" before marriage. Although the Bible is clear on the subject of intercourse outside of marriage, God is merciful and patient and He loves us unconditionally. I can also understand how the normal sex drives of two healthy people who love each other can cause an intense desire for sexual union. However, I'm even more convinced than before that it is God's desire for people to refrain from premarital intercourse and that obeying His instructions in this matter will be the very best for a relationship.

I came across this quote this past weekend. It's from *The Screwtape Letters* by C. S. Lewis: "The truth is that whenever a man lies with a woman, there, whether they like it or not, a transcendental relation is set up between them which must either be eternally enjoyed or eternally endured."[1] I can't think of anything more intimate or personal than sharing each other's bodies, emotions, and spirits in sexual union. That's why I'm so concerned about today's promiscuous sex. It's the philosophy of "easy come, easy go" or "if it feels good, do it." I know you agree with me that easy sex greatly cheapens intimacy. I know that this is not the situation in your case. You two love each other and are relatively committed to one another.

I've made up some questions that I hope you will discuss together. They may help you thoughtfully and carefully arrive at a decision to wait or not to wait. Keep in mind that I write these questions with the sense that you are both Christians who truly desire to grow in your Christian faith.

1. Will premarital intercourse lessen the meaning of intercourse in marriage for either of you? (Notice that in all these questions I'll include both of you in the decision-making process. I believe strongly that *both* of you must agree to this sexually active relationship. Otherwise the relationship will eventually be torn apart by bitterness and resentment.)

2. Does your conscience make you feel uneasy during or after sexual intercourse? This could be the Holy Spirit challenging you.

3. Are you both equally committed to each other?

4. Are you totally convinced in your hearts that the other person is "the one" forever?

5. What do you believe the Bible has to say about premarital sexual intercourse? Here are a few verses to look at: 1 Thessalonians 4:1-8; 1 Peter 2:11; 1 Corinthians 6:13, 18-20; Ephesians 5:3; and Acts 15:20.

6. You both seem to desire God's best for you. Will having sexual intercourse affect your usefulness to God or your relationship with Him?

7. Will having sexual intercourse before marriage damage in any way your relationship with each other?

8. Could premarital intercourse damage your communication or result in either a loss of respect for or mistrust of each other?

9. Will premarital intercourse help, hinder, or not affect your spiritual relationship to each other?

10. Have you thought through the possibilities of parenthood, marriage because of pregnancy, and birth control?

11. What are your motives for having sexual intercourse? Are they pure?

I'm convinced that any couple contemplating premarital intercourse should take a look at these questions and deal with them honestly.

I also want to include a list of statements for you to ponder. I found this list in an excellent book called *Sex, Love, or Infatuation: How Can I Really Know?* by Ray Short. In the chapter "To Be or Not To Be a Virgin," Ray writes that "science has established nine facts concerning the probable effect of premarital sex on your marriage."[2] I will list them for you. I wish I could include the whole chapter, but I'll simply list the statements. When you get together, you can discuss them as a couple. Don't be afraid to disagree with Ray or with each other. This will be a good exercise in communication and a great chance to learn a lot about premarital intercourse.

Fact 1. Premarital sex tends to break up couples.
Fact 2. Many men do not want to marry a woman

who has had intercourse with someone else.

Fact 3.  Those who have premarital sex tend to have less happy marriages.

Fact 4.  Those who have premarital sex are more likely to have their marriage end in divorce.

Fact 5.  Persons and couples who have had premarital sex are more likely to have extramarital affairs as well.

Fact 6.  Having premarital sex may fool you into marrying a person who is not right for you.

Fact 7.  Persons and couples with premarital sex experience seem to achieve sexual satisfaction sooner after they are married. HOWEVER—

Fact 8.  They are likely to be less satisfied overall with their sex life during marriage.[3]

To be honest, Ron and Tracy, I'm not sure where Ray Short got his information. But I think that each "fact" is worth your discussing. He has really made some important points for you to consider carefully.

The more I think about it, the more I respect you both for taking the time to consider what is best for you, for your relationship to each other, and for your relationship with God. I'm afraid too many couples simply move into intercourse too quickly. Without having given it much thought at all, they create a situation that can make a difference for their entire lives.

One last thing before I conclude. Even though right now you have little doubt that you probably will get married and of course don't want to think otherwise, let me play devil's advocate for a moment. Larry Richards says: "One study shows an average of five 'real loves' for kids between ninth grade and the second year of college."[4] You've both said that you have a long way to go before marriage. What if you don't get married? I know that I was thoroughly convinced I was going to marry Geri in junior high, Nancy in tenth grade, and Carol in twelfth grade! It's amazing how our minds can change!

I realize that I've given you a lot to think about. I believe in you both and look forward to spending more time together in the future. Thank you for the real privilege of being included in your life.

Your brother in Christ,

Jim

---

**Things to Think About**

• Do you think Ron and Tracy made the right decision to talk over their "big dilemma" with a counselor? Why or why not?

• What stands out in your mind from Jim's letter as being good advice?

• Which of the eleven questions that Jim asked Ron and Tracy were the most significant?

• What did you think of the nine scientific "facts" that Jim shared? Do you agree or disagree with them? Why?

• One study has shown that the average person has five "real loves" between ninth grade and the second year of college. Of course this is a general statement, but how does this statistic affect your opinion of teenage marriages?

---

# CHAPTER 4

# The Influence of Sexuality

One of the most powerful words in our language is that famous three-letter word "sex." Watch the next time you're with friends or at school. When the subject turns to sex, everyone stops to listen! One of the important questions everyone should consider is why sex has such an influence on our lives. A young friend of mine once made this comment about his own conversations: "With most of my friends, every subject we talk about gets turned into a talk about sex! Our society is sex crazy!"

Well, my high school friend was right. Our society is a little "sex crazy." I saw a T-shirt the other day that had printed in big red letters across the front, "Candy is dandy, but sex won't rot your teeth!" That's probably a true statement, but somehow I think there is more to the whole issue than that! And in order to better understand our sexuality, it's important to ask ourselves why sex does have such an important influence on our lives.

## The Media Appeals to Our Sexuality

Have you ever stopped to realize how frequently and effectively the media uses our sexuality to sell us products? Often you'll see a commercial on television where the most beautiful girl in the world is selling shaving cream, or Mr. World Universe with rippling muscles, wavy blond hair, a deep voice, and a golden tan tries to convince you that you, too, can look like he does if you would simply wear a certain cologne. And what's worse is that millions of us buy that brand of shaving cream or cologne because we fall for this media hype! (Believe me, it doesn't work. I've bought all that stuff and I'm still short and bald!) We are surrounded by sensual media, ranging from billboards to the latest love story at the theaters. And we have to face the fact that the media will always use the power of sexuality to get our attention.

## Sex is Mysterious

Another reason that sex has such an influence is that it's mysterious. I've been married more than nine years and sex is still a mystery! I'm not sure that there is a more profound mystery in the world. Every healthy person is curious about sex, and that's okay. When I speak at conferences and give the "sex talks," I'm always amazed at what a quiet and attentive audience I have. Is it because of my ability to communicate? I wish it were! It's because everyone is curious. Somehow we know that there is a beauty in the mystery of our sexuality. I think God made sex mysterious because He wanted us to keep it special. When sex quits being a mystery to you, that is the time to worry.

## Sex is Fun

Now this reason for sex being an influence in our lives might sound strange, but hear me out. Sex is fun. I can tell you from more than nine years of experience that sex is fun. God created sex to be enjoyable. I believe it gives Him great pleasure to provide His children with enjoyable experiences—and let's face it, sex is one of the all-time great experiences! Before you put the book down, read on . . .

One reason why people talk about sex so much is that it can be a wonderful experience. Don't be fooled, however, into thinking that all sex is fun. God wants the best for you, and that is why He asks you to save yourself for your marriage partner. And because premarital sexual intercourse is not what God intended for us, it often becomes anything but fun. I've met guys and girls who have had some negative sexual experiences and will bear the scars for their entire lives. Later I'll talk about sex outside of marriage. The main point I want to get across here is simply that we must be aware that sex is a major influence on our thinking.

No one will disagree that sex has an influence on our lives, but now it is important for us to take a serious look at another important question: "How does God view sex?" Most of you reading this book believe in God, most of you want to please Him, and most of you honestly want to live according to His will. In order to find out how God views sex and what His will is, we need to find out what the Bible says.

Many Christians need to erase certain ideas of what the Bible says about sex because, unfortunately, many of us were simply taught wrong! Well-meaning teachers communicated either directly or indirectly that sex is dirty, rotten, and ugly and that we should save this dirty, rotten, ugly experience for marriage. Please get this straight right now: God doesn't view your sexuality as dirty, rotten, or ugly!

God created your sexuality. Take a look at Genesis 2:18-25. It's the story of God creating Eve as a partner for Adam. Adam is ecstatic since the only companions he had before Eve were "all the beasts of the field and all

the birds of the air" (v. 19 RSV). They may be great for
pets, but they're not exactly what Adam had in mind for
a life-long partner. When Adam woke up from his little
nap and met Eve for the first time, he was excited. As the
Bible describes their relationship, it offers us a lesson:
"Therefore a man leaves his father and his mother and
cleaves to his wife, *and they become one flesh. And the
man and his wife were both naked, and were not
ashamed"* (Gen. 2:24-25 RSV, emphasis added).

God created man and woman. He created their
bodies, minds, and spirits. His hand was involved in
*every* aspect of their being, and their sexuality was a big
part of their being. Notice that when God created light,
darkness, the earth, vegetation, stars, birds, fish, and
animals, "God saw that it was good" (Gen. 1:1-25 RSV).
Yet when God made a partner for Adam, "it was *very*
good" (Gen. 1:31 RSV, emphasis added).

In my opinion, any view other than the belief that
God created our sexuality and that He sees it as *very*
good is a warped view. The problem with our society's
attitude toward sex is that it is incomplete. Since our
sexuality was created by God, we should view it as His
special gift to us.

Let's take a look at another passage from the Bible,
this time from the New Testament:

Flee from sexual immorality. All other sins a man
commits are outside his body, but he who sins sexually sins against his own body. Do you not know
that your body is a temple of the Holy Spirit, who is
in you, whom you have received from God? You are
not your own; you were bought at a price. Therefore
honor God with your body. (1 Cor. 6:18-20 RSV)

When I read this section of God's word, a couple of
points really jump off the page. First, our bodies are
temples of God. The Holy Spirit of God actually dwells
within our bodies. I take this to mean that our bodies are

special and that we should treat them with respect and honor. This is true as we deal with our sexuality, decide how much we eat, or work on keeping our "temples" in shape physically.

The other point that jumps out of this passage is that we are to glorify God with our bodies. What you do with your body is one of the few things in life that is almost totally under your own control. You must choose whether to honor God or to dishonor Him with your body. A decision you make about sexual relations may or may not honor your Lord.

Let's face it. Throughout our entire lives—even at retirement—sex will influence us. The big question for you and me is *how* it will influence us. Make sure that you question the media's influence. Make sure that you learn what God's desire for your sexuality is all about. Then you'll never have to settle for a counterfeit love.

---

### Things to Think About

• The media is mentioned as a major influence on our thinking about sex. Do you agree or disagree? Why?

• What are specific ways to keep the strong sexual influence of the media out of our lives?

• If God created sex and sees it as very good, why would He ask us to wait until marriage to have sexual intercourse?

• Why do you think the world is so interested in sex?

---

The *Handling Your Hormones* growth guide can help you further understand the influence of society and God's standards for us.

# CHAPTER 5

# Sexual Intercourse

People have described intercourse as
"thrilling, soul-stirring, boring, shock-
ing, deeply satisfying, painful, wonderfully comfortable,
disappointing, fascinating, disgusting, delightful"—and
the list could go on and on.[1] That's why, when teenagers
were asked the question, "What subjects do you wish
you knew more about?" in a survey about sexuality, the
number one answer was sexual intercourse.[2]

This same survey also tells us that nearly 6 out of 10
16-18-year-olds have had sexual intercourse.[3] This
means that not only are people wanting information
about sexual intercourse *before* they experience it, but
that they are also interested *after* they've experienced it.
We can conclude, too, that people may have sexual
intercourse without understanding it. I think it is healthy
to want to learn about and to wonder about sexual intercourse. Wondering what it would be like with your husband or wife is definitely not nasty. In fact, it is very, very
normal.

Wondering about sexual intercourse can lead us to
want to know what God says about it. We may find that
there aren't as many do's and don'ts as we sometimes
think. The Bible clearly states, however, that sexual intercourse outside of marriage is not right in God's eyes.
You've probably heard the words "adultery" and "forni-

and "fornication." Here is how *Webster's New Collegiate Dictionary* defines them. Adultery is "voluntary sexual intercourse between a married man and someone other than his wife or between a married woman and someone other than her husband." Fornication is "human sexual intercourse other than between a man and his wife: sexual intercourse between a spouse and an unmarried person: sexual intercourse between unmarried people."

As a high school student who had recently become a Christian, I had numerous questions about sexuality and I was frustrated because at times the Bible didn't seem clear enough. At other times I questioned why the Bible seemed so old-fashioned in not allowing intercourse before marriage. Is God the great kill-joy when it comes to sexuality? Many people reading this book have similar questions. I want to help answer some of these questions by stating four reasons for sexual intercourse in marriage. These four reasons are not necessarily in any order; each one is, however, an important dimension of the role intercourse has in marriage.

### Unity: One Flesh

In a mysterious, almost sacred sense, when two people have sexual intercourse they become one flesh. Even the physical act of inserting the penis into the vagina is symbolic of the oneness and unity of the couple. The Bible puts it this way: "Therefore a man leaves his father and his mother and cleaves to his wife, *and they become one flesh*" (Gen. 2:24 RSV, emphasis added). This verse speaks of a real oneness in which a couple is so intimate that each person completely shares the other's nakedness. Interestingly, the next verse in Genesis says, "the man and his wife were both naked, and were not ashamed" (Gen. 2:25 RSV). This idea of unity as one flesh is seldom talked about today, yet it is a very special aspect of sexual intercourse.

## Communication

Perhaps the deepest form of communication and love is intercourse. I am constantly reminded, during intercourse with my wife, that we are physically expressing and sharing our deepest love for one another. There is a certain tender feeling during this intimate experience that communicates a sense of unconditional love similar to the sacrificial love that God has for humankind. During intercourse, you are communicating the deepest sense of commitment. Intercourse only for selfish pleasure is second-rate at best; in fact, it subtly communicates a strong message of disregard for the other person that can be quite hurtful.

## Enjoyment

As I said in a previous chapter, sex is fun! In my opinion, there is nothing more enjoyable in all the world than the mutually shared experience of marital sexual intercourse. In a recent counseling session, a sixteen-year-old girl was talking about her problems. Referring to her first intercourse experience, she said, "I didn't enjoy it all. It was rushed, I was afraid, and the car was uncomfortable." That is *not* how intercourse was meant to be. Intercourse was meant to be experienced in the relaxed, romantic, leisurely atmosphere of the marriage bed—not in the back seat of a Datsun!

I feel sorry for the Puritans of our country in the late 1600s. Many of them actually believed that the only reason for sexual intercourse was "making babies." They were correct that intercourse can create another life, but it can be so much more than an act of procreation. The pure enjoyment, the intimate communication, and the symbolic and physical oneness of married intercourse make it one of the most special gifts God has ever given humankind.

## Procreation

Of course, intercourse is God's method of creating a child. It is a miracle designed by God. And I consider it one of His all-time greatest miracles and an all-around wonderful idea! The miracle of a male's sperm making contact with the female's egg at precisely the right time to create life is an incredible occurrence! The beauty of two married people who love each other very much helping God create another life, blood of their blood, flesh of their flesh, is beyond the written or spoken word.

God's special purpose in creating sex was that two married people would produce an offspring from their own lives. It is a tragedy that more than a million *unwanted* pregnancies happen each year. It is a shame that something as wonderful as creating new life is taken so lightly by so many people in our generation. When two people believe that they are mature enough to have sexual intercourse, they should think through the eventual possibility of raising a child as husband and wife. If they haven't dealt with the issue of parenting, they haven't experienced intercourse as God intended humankind to experience it.

Having explored the Scriptures regarding premarital or extramarital intercourse, I no longer view God as the great kill-joy. I understand that when you create something as special and meaningful as the intimacy of sexual intercourse, you are wanting the very best for your creation. God knew that the best sex is sex shared by a man and a woman who love each other unconditionally and who are committed to making their relationship last a lifetime through marriage. I'm not saying that all sexual intercourse outside of marriage produces only negative feelings. I'd be lying to you if I said that. Instead, I'm saying, "Why settle for second best when God's way brings the true fulfillment that sexual intercourse was designed to produce?"

---

### Things to Think About

• Do the teenagers you know wish they had more information about sexual intercourse?

• What other subjects in the area of sexuality do you think teenagers want more information about?

• Do you think Jim was right to include "enjoyment" as one of the reasons for sexual intercourse? Why or why not?

• Do you agree or disagree with this statement on procreation: "When two people believe they are mature enough to have sexual intercourse, they should think through the eventual possibility of raising a child as husband and wife. If they haven't dealt with the issue of parenting, they haven't experienced intercourse as God intended humankind to experience it." Give reasons for your answer.

---

# CHAPTER 6

# Differences in the Way Men and Women Respond

Guys can be such perverts! All my boy-friend ever thinks about is sex. I'm not a prude, but I really want to know if there are guys in this world who think about anything other than sex!" I get a question like this at every seminar I teach on sex. And the answer to this girl's question is yes *and* no. Of course guys think about things other than sex. But most healthy adolescent boys can easily spend a lot of time thinking about sex.

It seems to me that besides the obvious physical dif-ferences between male and female human beings, there are some other significant differences that are important to discuss—and the question above points to one such difference. You can attribute these differences to biology, cultural conditioning, or whatever you like, but acknowl-edging some of these basic differences might help you understand why your special friend acts the way he or she does.

Many experts in the field of sex and dating say that one critical difference between the male and female has to do with the relationship of sex and love. Josh McDo-well, a popular Christian speaker, says, "I'm convinced sex is more dominant in the mind of a man, and love is more paramount in the mind of a woman."[1] When a couple goes to a romantic movie, often the male thinks

"sex" and the female thinks "love." After the first romantic scene, the male is ready to park on Inspiration Point
and miss the rest of the movie. The female responds
more to the idea of love and the beauty of romance. The
female is much more interested in the love story while
the male is more interested in a replay of the action—
now!

As you can see, like Josh McDowell, I'm convinced
that the subject of sex is more often dominant in the
minds of guys and love is more often dominant in the
minds of girls. It's not that girls aren't interested in sex or
guys in love, but there is a difference. Perhaps the difference stems from what stimulates (or turns on) a guy and
a girl. A guy is usually ready for sex any time, any place,
at a moment's notice. A girl, on the other hand, is stimulated by romantic movies, flowers, a slight touch on the
shoulder. Guys are stimulated by sight, girls by touch. Of
course I'm speaking in generalities!

Guys can be sexually aroused in a matter of sec-
onds. (I'm serious!) It takes girls longer. I've often com-
pared a male's sex drive to a drum solo by your favorite
rock band. The male sex drive is intense. It builds quickly
to a climax, explodes with excitement, and then ends as
quickly as it started. A woman's sex drive is more like a
Bach concerto. It takes a little longer to get going. It
builds to a tremendous climax, slowly settles down, and
then ends softly. Why do I mention these differences? To
help you understand and perhaps think more carefully
about your actions when it comes to sexual stimulation.

If, for instance, you girls could only understand what
you are doing to us guys with what you wear or don't
wear! Remember, a guy is stimulated by sight. Now I'm
not recommending turtleneck sweaters or ankle-length
gowns for the beach. I am advising, however, that when
you get dressed for a date you remember that what you
are wearing can definitely help create a mood and

atmosphere for the date.

I'm convinced that most of the time girls just do not think about or even realize what they are doing to guys when they dress in certain ways. I'll never forget a time when sixteen of us traveled by houseboat for a week. The first night a number of the girls came into the kitchen to visit us guys as we were playing a game at the table. The girls were wearing long T-shirts and bikini panties—and that was it. No bras and nothing over the panties. After the girls moved on through the kitchen, the guys went absolutely crazy. Their minds had definitely shifted from concentrating on the game to thoughts about something else!

I decided not to make a big deal of it, but to talk to the girls about what turns guys on. The next day we had a wonderful talk. I'm convinced that those girls simply had not thought that what they were wearing would turn those guys on. When it comes to how a girl dresses or acts around guys, she must continually think through how guys react, especially if she wants to steer clear of trouble.

Guys also need to be careful about what they wear and what they say and do. Girls are attracted by sight, but they are also attracted by touch and talk. Guys need to be careful about what they say to girls. I have a friend who told his girlfriend on the second date that he loved her. The problem was that she believed him! She fell madly and passionately in love with him. When he saw what those powerful three words did to her, he backed down and tried to explain: "I really didn't mean 'love'!"

I guess what I'm trying to say is that males and females respond differently when it comes to sexuality. Of course, there are also many similarities in their responses, but one of the smartest things you can do is to be aware of the basic differences. Think through your actions and avoid any position that might cause frustration to others. Once you're sensitive to these differences between men and women, you needn't be threatened by them. You may even be able to see how these differences enrich your relationships with members of the opposite sex.

---

**Things to Thing About**

• Do you agree that, in general, guys are more motivated by sex and girls more motivated by love?
• What things do you think girls do or wear that stimulate guys?
• What things do you think guys do or wear that stimulate girls?
• Do you think it is important to understand some of the differences between males and females? Why or why not?

---

# CHAPTER 7

# How to Know If You Are in Love

Recently I watched a group of high school girls on the beach check out a handsome lifeguard. (Who says guys are the only ones who look at the scenery on the beach?) As the lifeguard leisurely walked to the water to cool off, the girls went crazy with excitement! One of the girls making the most noise sighed and exclaimed, "I've never seen such a fox! I think I'm in love!"

I don't think her reaction was unusual—in fact, it was quite normal. I even remember saying very similar words when I was in high school and college. (Not about male lifeguards, of course!) Let's think about the girl's remarks, though. The lifeguard may have been a fox, but I doubt that the girl was really "in love." She was "in infatuation." She was attracted to this young lifeguard on a physical level. Perhaps she even had a fantasy of walking hand in hand with him down the beach at sunset. But was she "in love"? Not at all.

I remember my first crush on a girl. Her name was Geri. She was absolutely beautiful. I was totally convinced that someday we would walk down the aisle together. I think I liked her most because she was a better baseball player than I was and she was also the only girl in elementary school who would play sports with us guys! I liked her for years. In fact, once in junior high school, I wrote a note to her and signed it with "I love you." From that day on she hardly ever talked to me! I think I scared her away. Was that love? No, it was infatuation. It was what is sometimes called "puppy love."

Infatuation is a normal part of life. Infatuation involves many of the same emotions and feelings that real love does. The major difference between love and infatuation is that real love stands the test of time.

From the moment I met Cathy (the woman who is now my wife) I was attracted to her. In fact, I was infatuated with her. I knew that I loved her, though, when I was still attracted to her after two and a half years of dating. Furthermore, I was *committed* to her. When I first met her, I had never imagined that she had the normal human faults that everyone else has. I imagined that she and our relationship were perfect. As time went on, I saw otherwise. Neither of us was (or is) perfect. The relationship wasn't perfect, and it wasn't always easy. When even after an argument I still cared deeply for Cathy, then I knew that this was becoming more than infatuation. Real love stands the test of disagreements and of time.

There is no easy way to determine whether you are in love for keeps or not. If you are a teenager, something to think about is a statistic I've already mentioned: it is quite possible that you will "fall in love" about five different times between the ninth grade and your second year of college. As a teenager, you will experience different degrees of love, but the odds are against you marrying your high-school sweetheart and living happily ever after. I'm not saying that it doesn't happen. I am saying that the statistical odds are against it happening.

As I said before, there are no simple answers to the important question, "How do I know I'm in love?" I do, however, want to give you a few practical guidelines to help you decide if a particular person might be "the one"!

### 1. Are You Willing to Give 100 Percent of Yourself to Your Mate?

Do you believe your mate is willing to give 100 percent of himself or herself to you? True love is selfless love. Even when you are tired or have had a bad day, selfless love will enable you to meet the needs of your partner. A selfish love grows old quickly when its own needs are not being met.

### 2. Do You *Like* the Other Person?

I'll never forget a scene in the movie *Shenandoah*. One young man approached another man to ask for his daughter's hand in marriage. The father asked, "Do you like my daughter?" The young man answered, "I love your daughter!" The wise old father said, "I didn't ask you if you loved her. I asked you 'Do you like her?'"

Sometimes people get married even though they don't really like the personality or behavior of their partner. Often they think they'll change the other person. This plan is rarely successful. So ask yourself if you like your partner even with his or her faults. And consider, too, whether you could live with his or her faults. And consider, too, whether you could live with those faults forever!

### 3. Are You Transparent with Each Other?

Is your relationship one in which you can be open and honest with each other? Open communication is one of the major tools in a positive relationship. I've never seen a good relationship that didn't have this element of transparency.

## 4. Are You and Your Special Friend Too Dependent on Each Other?

There are two different types of relationships: "I love, therefore I need" and "I need, therefore I love." The second type can be a real loser in the long run. Many relationships, however, are based on this "I need, therefore I love" idea, and these usually end up down the drain. Either one person ceases to "need" and therefore ceases to "love," or the other person gets tired of this total dependency and eventually leaves.

## 5. Is Your Love Self-Centered?

When a person is infatuated with someone, that person is often asking, "What's in this for me?" This type of love involves *getting* rather than *giving*. A self-centered love is not a true love; it is counterfeit love. Our goal in love should be what the Greeks termed *agape* love. This is a love with no strings attached. It's the same type of self-giving, self-sacrificing love that God has for you.

## 6. Do You Have a Mature Love for Jesus Christ?

I believe that a good test of true love is to ask if both people involved can honestly say, "I have a desire to be all that God wants me to be. I am willing to put the Lord Jesus Christ first in my own life and in my friend's life. Our relationship to each other is second to my relationship to Christ." The couples I know who are really doing well are those who have a good relationship with God individually and together as a couple. A love that is tied together with the love of God is the strongest kind of love.

I would suggest that you take a good hard look at the type of love Paul talks about in 1 Corinthians 13. The qualities of love he describes in his "love chapter" can be a measuring stick to help you examine if you really are in love. When reading this chapter, look especially at the qualities of love in verses 4-7 (NIV):

> Love is patient, love is kind. It does not envy, it does not boast, it is not proud. It is not rude, it is not self-seeking, it is not easily angered, it keeps no record of wrongs. Love does not delight in evil but rejoices with the truth. It always protects, always trusts, always hopes, always perseveres.

This definition of love which Paul offers us here can help us honestly evaluate our love for another person.

Love is a uniquely wonderful experience. Unfortunately the genuine experience of love can be closely imitated by an experience of infatuation. As time passes and presents us with storms to weather and new perspectives on our lives, we can then better distinguish between infatuation and real love. Right now, I think it could be important for you to deal with the questions that I present here, study the ideals of love which Paul sets forth, and trust God to show you His desire for your special relationship. And, as trite as it sounds, time is on your side.

---

**Things to Think About**

• What are some differences between love and infatuation?

• Do you think most students are experiencing love or infatuation?

• Is infatuation wrong? Why or why not?

• Read over 1 Corinthians 13:4-7. What impresses you about these qualities of love?

_____

Further questions in the *Handling Your Hormones* growth guide may help you determine whether you are "in love" or "in infatuation."

# CHAPTER 8

# Unconditional Love

Once upon a time there was a young girl named Susie. She was a beautiful little girl with the most wonderful doll collection in the world. Her father traveled all over the world on business, and for nearly twelve years he had brought dolls home to Susie. In her bedroom she had shelves of dolls from all over the United States and from every continent on earth. She had dolls that could sing and dance and do just about anything a doll could possibly do.

One day one of her father's business acquaintances came to visit. During dinner he asked Susie about her wonderful doll collection. After they ate, Susie took him by the hand and showed him these marvelous dolls from all over the world. He was very impressed. After he took the "grand tour" and was introduced to many of the beautiful dolls, he asked Susie, "With all these precious dolls, you must have one that is your favorite. Which one is it?"

Without a moment's hesitation Susie went over to her old beat-up toy box and started pulling out toys. From the bottom of the box she pulled out one of the most ragged dolls you have ever seen. There were only a few strands of hair left on its head. The clothing had long since disappeared. The doll was filthy from many years of playing outside. One of the buttons for the eyes was hanging down with only a string to keep it connected. Stuffing was coming out at the elbow and knee. Susie handed the doll to the gentleman and said, "This is my favorite."

The man was shocked and asked, "Why this doll, with all these beautiful dolls in your room?"

Susie replied, "If I didn't love this doll, nobody would!"

That simple statement moved the businessman to tears. It was simple yet very profound. The little girl loved her doll unconditionally. She loved the doll not for its beauty or abilities but simply because it was her very own doll.

In this same way, God loves you unconditionally, not for what you do but for who you are. You are His child. Millions of people in the world miss the simple fact that they are loved unconditionally by God. God accepts you. He believes in you and He wants the best for you.

Sometimes we feel that we don't deserve God's love. Sometimes we can't understand how God could have such patience with us when we continually mess up. Well, listen to this: *God's ways are different from our ways.* He doesn't love you only if you do certain things or live a certain life-style. He loves you—period! When people finally understand the depth of God's love, they are free to be all that He wants them to be. Interestingly, people who comprehend this unconditional love have an easier time staying away from the sin that can clog their relationship with God.

A perfect illustration of God's unconditional love is found in the story of the Prodigal Son which Jesus told in Luke 15:11-24. The parable opens with a father's younger son asking for his share of his father's property. Receiving half of the estate, the young man then goes to a distant country and proceeds to squander the wealth. Soon finding himself without a penny to his name in a country struck by a famine, the boy returns to his father's home. His father sees him from a distance and runs to greet him with open arms. The son's first words are, "Father, I have sinned against heaven and against you. I am no longer worthy to be called your son" (v. 21 NIV). The father's joyful reaction to his son's return, however, is to feast and celebrate because, in this loving father's words, "this son of mine was dead and is alive again; he was lost and is found" (v. 24 NIV).

The son definitely sinned against his father. He wasted his money on "wild living." Yet look at what happened when the son asked to come home as a hired hand! The father realized how the son had sinned, but he took his son back with open arms. The father joyfully celebrated the return of his wayward boy.

The reason that this story is so fitting in a book on sex is that many of us have had a little trouble handling our hormones. We've slipped from the biblical standard of sexuality. At times we've even turned our backs on God and gone our own way. But the good news is that, no matter what we've done or how we've strayed, God waits for us with open arms. He loves all His children and nothing in the world makes Him happier than for one of His children to wise up and come back to Him. Be assured that when we do go to Him, He receives us with a depth of love beyond human comprehension.

Before leaving this topic, let's review a few facts about the unconditional love of God.


**God Loves You Not for What You Do But for Who You Are**

Sometimes this concept is very difficult to understand, but it is very true that you are deeply loved by God. He created you and He loves His creation. Even if you have turned your back on Him, He is there, like the father in the story of the Prodigal Son, with open arms and warm acceptance. Remember, too, that the Christian faith is not based on rules and regulations; the Christian faith is based on a relationship between God and you. And remember that God never changes this desire to have a relationship with you, no matter what you do. When a person understands that God's love is not contingent on our actions, that person's life can be radically different.

## God's Ways Are Different from Our Ways

One of the reasons we have so much trouble accepting God's love is that it is often contrary to what we know on a human level. In life we must often *earn* acceptance by trying out for the baseball team or getting good grades or measuring up to some standards, either real or imagined. But God's love is there no matter what we do or don't do. God loves the drunk sleeping in the gutter in New York City as much as He loves you, and He loves Billy Graham or Mother Teresa no more than He loves you. God cherishes each one of His creations.

## God Loves You Sacrificially

God's deep and piercing love for you cost Him the life of His only Son. The ultimate sacrifice of Jesus dying on the Cross so that you might have abundant life on earth and eternal life afterwards is the greatest demonstration of love that the world has ever known. The apostle Paul put it this way: "But God demonstrates his own love for us in this: While we were still sinners, Christ died for us" (Rom. 5:9 NIV).

## The Gift of God's Love Is Free

All you have to do is accept God's gift of love. One of the hardest things in life is to accept love we feel we don't deserve, but when we do, we can't help but be transformed by God's unconditional and overflowing love for us. As we begin to realize that we are loved despite our mistakes, this deep love will draw us even closer to God.

---

## Things to Think About

- How did you react to the story of Susie and her doll collection?
- Why do you think people have such a difficult time accepting God's unconditional love?
- Can you relate to the story of the Prodigal Son mentioned in this chapter? If so, how?
- Do you think it was important to include a chapter on unconditional love in this book? Why or why not?

---

# CHAPTER 9

# Peer Pressure

No one is exempt from peer pressure. This demand to conform to a particular group or to society in general is made on people of all ages. The pressure to conform comes in various shapes and sizes. Sometimes it is subtle; sometimes it is blatant. No one with a heartbeat, though, can say that he or she has never had to battle peer pressure.

Peer pressure can often be a spiritual dilemma involving the battle between the spirit and the flesh (the sinful nature in all of us). If you for one moment think that you are the only one fighting this battle, you're wrong. Even the apostle Paul suffered deeply from this war within. Listen to him talk about his struggle:

I do not understand what I do. For what I want to do I do not do, but what I hate I do . . . . I know that nothing good lives in me, that is, in my sinful nature. For I have the desire to do what is good, but I cannot carry it out. For what I do is not the good I want to do; no, the evil I do not want to do—this I keep on doing. Now if I do what I do not want to do, it is no longer I who do it, but it is sin living in me that does it. (Rom. 7:15, 18-20 NIV)

I think Paul was a lot like you and me. He made mistakes and he often missed the mark, but by no means was he an evil person. His deepest desire was to do right.

He didn't want to settle for second best, but at times he blew it. His insight about his failings was brilliant. He was able to see this problem for what it actually was—*a spiritual battle*. He really did want to do right, yet he kept messing up. At the end of his little discourse he answered his own question: "Who will rescue me from this body of death? Thanks be to God—through Christ Jesus our Lord!" (Rom. 7:25 NIV). For Paul, the solution to the problem of being pressured to conform to the world's standards came from Jesus Christ. Paul didn't spiritualize the issue and tell his readers that his problems were over forever. He simply knew *who* would help him in the battle.

You can be assured that temptations will come and go, but like Paul you can be confident that God will help you work through the temptations when you seek His help. In fact, Paul wrote to a group of people in the city of Corinth and said,

No temptation has seized you except what is common to man. And God is faithful; he will not let you be tempted beyond what you can bear. But when you are tempted, he will also provide a way out so that you can stand up under it. (1 Cor. 10:13 NIV)

In Christ you have the power to deal with peer pressure. Here are a few suggestions that can make the battle a little easier.

### Don't Let Peer Pressure Sneak Up on You

Use your head! Know when you are being pressured to conform to a standard that is second-best! Face the pressure and carefully think about the possible outcome of your action. Ask questions like these: "Am I settling for second best?," "Will my actions be pleasing to God?," "Am I being pressured to do something that I feel isn't right?" Sometimes by thinking logically and looking at all the options, we can find it easier to overcome a temptation.

## Remember That Everyone You Spend Time with Has an Influence on You

It always fascinates me when I watch groups or cliques of people hanging around with each other. If one person in the group likes a certain type of music, usually the others will also like that type of music. If one person wears a certain style of clothes, others in the group will probably wear that same style. Our friends play an important part in determining who we are, what we stand for, and where we are going in life. That's why it is important to choose our friends wisely.

God's Word has much to say about friends and companions. Proverbs 22:24-25, for instance, offers us this lesson: "Do not make friends with a hot-tempered man, do not associate with one easily angered, or you may learn his ways and get yourself ensnared" (NIV). It's all too easy to pick up bad habits from friends. On the other hand, the right kind of friends can influence us toward bettering our lives: "As iron sharpens iron, so one man sharpens another" (Prov. 27:17 NIV).

Perhaps you need to take an inventory of your friends. Ask yourself:

• Are my friends a positive or a negative influence on my life?

• Are my friends helping me to be all that God wants me to be, or are they tearing me down?

• What kind of influence do my friends have on my life?

If your answers show you that your friends are a negative influence, it is time to make some major decisions about your friendships. Remember that "He who walks with the wise grows wise, but a companion of fools suffers harm" (Prov. 13:20 NIV).

### Choose Your Friends Wisely

I had a friend named Bob. We used to talk for hours. He had a strong desire to do right. He wanted to be a professional baseball player, he wanted to get good grades, and he wanted to be a "success with the girls." Bob also had a strong desire to be a growing Christian. He would talk and fantasize about baseball and these other dreams, yet he never seemed to achieve any of his goals. He was always falling down and failing.

Finally, after months of struggling, Bob offered me an insight into his problems when he told me about his "flaky friends" and how they would always bring him down. I said, "You know, it's your choice to be so influenced by those friends. Why don't you spend a little less time with them and a little more time with Robert and Doug?" Bob had told me earlier that Robert and Doug were very good influences on him.

Bob took my advice. He still spent time with his old "flaky" friends, but he began to *choose* to spend more and more time with Robert and Doug. You can guess what happened. Every area of his life began to improve. Because of Robert and Doug's influence, Bob was motivated to get his act together. Bob couldn't kick the negative influence of peer pressure on his own, but he chose to be influenced by positive peer pressure. And that made all the difference for him.

### Remember Your Uniqueness: You Are Special in God's Eyes

Never forget that *God loves you for who you are, not*

*for what you do.* You are a special person in God's eyes. Because of His unconditional love, you are free to be all that He created you to be! Consider, too, that Jesus said, "You will know the truth, and the truth will set you free" (John 8:32 NIV). A person who truly understands that he or she is loved by God will not be as motivated to conform to peer pressure. He or she instead understands what it is to be accepted by the One whose acceptance is truly important: God Himself.

### Seek First the Kingdom of God

In the midst of our daily activities and responsibilities, it is easy to get distracted. Jesus gave us some sound advice when He said, "But seek first his kingdom and his righteousness, and all these things will be given to you as well" (Matt. 6:33 NIV). If we put God first, He will provide the necessities of life. Unfortunately, we often worry more about what people think than about what God wants for us.

An important factor in overcoming the pull of negative peer pressure is the possession of the inner strength that comes with a healthy self-image. When you put God first in your life, you can develop that stronger self-image. After all, you were created in *His* image! And even though you are flawed by sin, He values you so much that He sent Christ to die for you. As you develop this improved self-image, you gain inner strength and then you are better able to say no to peer pressure.

Interestingly enough, the people I know who overcome peer pressure are people who are more concerned about seeking God than they are about pleasing their friends. They are seeking first His kingdom. In fact, as they do that, they seem to have better relationships with their friends than anyone else I know.

### It's Hard to Say No

Another topic related to peer pressure and sex and dating is the "it's hard to say no" problem. Many, many young people have been pressured into experiencing sex when they really didn't want to—simply because they didn't know how to say no. I've talked to a number of people who have really regretted not saying "no thanks" before it was too late.

In his book on teenage sexuality, Aaron Haas reports the results of his survey of teenagers' sexual attitudes. His findings on the subject of "saying no" are very enlightening. Teenagers were asked, for instance, "Have there been times when you have been on a date, when you had sexual contact even though you really did not feel like it?" Forty-three percent of the guys who were fifteen and sixteen and a whopping 65 percent of the girls of the same age answered yes. Nearly half of the guys and more than half of the girls who were fifteen and sixteen have had a difficult time saying "No thanks."[1]

What were the reasons these young people gave for acting contrary to their true feelings? Here are some of the answers and circumstances explained to Dr. Haas:

"I didn't want to hurt his/her feelings."
"I didn't want him/her to think I was a prude!"
"I really felt pressured."
"I just couldn't say 'No'!"
"I was afraid that he/she wouldn't like me if I said 'No'!"
"I don't know why, but I felt obligated to go along with him/her."
"I was high" or "I was drunk!"
"It meant a lot to him and not much to me."
"I didn't want to seem like a tease."
"I was afraid she would think I didn't like her."

"I wanted to prove I was a man."
"I did it for the experience."
"There was nothing else to do."[2]

These statements show that at times many people can feel insecure. They, too, can be afraid to say no. They don't want to hurt someone's feelings. I think, however, that any boyfriend or girlfriend who is worth keeping will greatly respect your ability to say "no thanks." If the other person is only interested in your body, then he or she isn't worth keeping. It really is hard to say no, but it's always worth it.

Before concluding this chapter, I want to list a few of the lines guys and girls use on each other. In print they look absurd, but in the heat of passion they seem to make sense. When sexual feelings are running high, even the most honest person may become desperate and try to manipulate another person. Although there is probably a line for every day of the year, I'll mention only a few of the key ideas that seem to be used year after year.

• "It's okay if we both agree to do it."
Usually one person in a relationship is more eager to have sexual intercourse than the other is. If he or she can get the other person to agree verbally, then that seems to make the action okay.

• "You're the only person I will ever love, so let's not wait until we are married."
This argument is powerful, but usually it simply isn't true. The average person has at least five loves during the teenage years and early twenties. Since this statement about loving one person is usually false, it's a ridiculous line for a person to use—especially if he claims to love the person he's talking to.

• "If you really love me . . . "
This is the "you've got to prove your love to me" line: "If you really love me, prove it." This line is most successfully used by "macho" older guys who are dating younger girls. Sometimes a person with a poor self-image falls for this line also.

• "Let's experiment to see what it's like. If we don't like it, we'll never have to do it again."
People actually fall for this! The aggressor knows that if the partner gives approval once, he or she will most likely give in again at other times. Remember that it's harder to say no the second time.

• "Everybody's doing it. Are you a square?"
First let me say, "Wrong! Everybody isn't doing it!" On any junior high, high school, or college campus there are people who have chosen not to be sexually active— and often they are the real leaders in the school. You are not a square if you choose not to engage in sexual promiscuity. You are a square if you succumb to peer pressure because of a flimsy line like this one!

• "If it happens, it happens!"
These words are usually said by the person who is always bringing up the subject of sex. Be careful of people who are always raising philosophical questions about sex, asking personal questions about your sex life, and keeping the subject before you so much that it would be easy to be tempted. This line is a sly one but it works—just ask thousands of disappointed girls and guys who fell for it.

Peer pressure is real. It's a fact of life which we all must deal with at any age, but the pressure seems much more difficult to deal with at certain times of our lives. I know that peer pressure combined with a poor self-image and a deep love for another person can cause us to do things we might later regret. We can deal with this pressure more easily when we choose friends who will be supportive of us. It also helps to spend time considering God's love for us. Trust in this love and rely on God's promises to be with you as you face temptations and pressure from your peers.

---

### Things to Think About

• Why is it so difficult to fight the battle of peer pressure?

• Why do you think so many people have such a problem saying no to sex even when they don't want to have it?

• Do you agree or disagree with the idea that the people you spend time with have a profound influence on you? Why?

• What makes you unique in God's eyes?

---

# CHAPTER 10

# Dating

I can always tell when the high school prom is about to take place. Many of the girls in my youth group begin to feel extremely depressed. It's the Sunday before the big dance and it looks like they'll be spending another prom night at the movies with their girlfriends who also weren't asked to the prom. To tell you the truth, I'm beginning to resent proms because of all the damage they do to the self-images and emotions of my young friends. It is a shame that an event that draws only about 25 percent of the school's population can do so much damage to so many of those not attending.

This emphasis on the prom brings into focus the fact that the great American institution—the date—is going as strong as ever. For many of us, dating is a great paradox. Most people dream of the perfect, romantic date. Most young people can hardly wait to start dating. Dating can be great fun. It can be all you ever dreamed about. But the paradox is that dating can also cause more distress, hurt feelings, and self-doubt than just about anything else I've ever seen. Before we deal with some helpful advice, I want to clear up two misunderstandings about dating.

**Misunderstanding #1:** *Almost everybody dates in high school.*

Wrong. Statistics tell us that 50 percent of the girls and 40 percent of the guys graduating from high school have *never* dated. If you happen to fall into this category, you are definitely not alone. Here's a note a youth volunteer gave me on the back of a church bulletin one time after I shared this statistic at a youth meeting: "Thanks, Jim, for letting our kids know that not everyone dates in high school. The biggest problem in my life was that I didn't date in high school. I thought I was the only one. I hated myself, my looks, my personality, my church—everything. Years later I realized how grateful I was for being a 'late bloomer.' I was able to establish positive high school friendships that have lasted a lifetime and I have a wonderful husband I met while in college. I wish I'd heard your talk years ago."

Here's an excerpt from another letter with a different perspective on the same issue: "I wish I hadn't dated at such a young age. I didn't know how to handle my emotions. I let guys use me. Of course I wasn't aware of this at the time. But now, after two abortions, I wish I hadn't grown up so fast . . . . "

**Misunderstanding #2:** *If you want to be popular, you must be sexually active.*
Again, this is simply wrong. *Everybody isn't doing it!* Of the high schoolers who were elected to Who's Who Among American High School Students in 1982, 73 percent had never had sexual relations. If you could survey some of the popular people at your school, you would find out that not everyone is sexually active. Yes, they have a normal sex drive and curiosity and all the rest, but they recognize that they must deal with other more important priorities.

One of the finest compliments I've ever heard was a statement by a young girl in our youth group. She was telling me about one of our high school seniors whom she described like this: "John is cute, he's popular at school, and he's so involved in sports. I love being around him because he's so together, and if you can believe this, he is still a virgin!"

I think my young friend was amazed that a person could be cute, popular, and "together" and still *choose* to be a virgin. There are, in fact, thousands of people who have chosen as an act of their will *not* to be sexually active and who still seem to have a lot of friends and a certain degree of popularity.

A few things I've said are worth repeating. First, it isn't true that everybody dates in high school. Second, it isn't necessary to be sexually active in order to be popular. Dating can be fun and your time for dating will come. Whether that time is now or in the future, I have some suggestions for you.

### Establish a Friendship

As I shared earlier, the first day I saw the woman who is now my wife, I fell deeply "in infatuation" with her. She didn't know I existed, but I knew it was "infatuation at first sight." Back then I might have said "*love* at first sight" but now I know better. Anyway, I'll never forget that day in the campus gym . . .

I was at freshman orientation with two other new-comers to the college whom I had met at dinner. Cathy was being entertained by a group of upperclassmen who seemed to have some of the same feelings I had! I leaned over to my two freshman friends, pointed Cathy out to them, and said, "See that girl over there? I'm going to take her out some time." They looked at her, they looked at me, and they laughed. They thought I was kidding, but I wasn't.

I was lucky enough to have the same English class and psychology class that Cathy had. It just so happened that I would try to sit next to her whenever I could manage it—which was pretty often since I would wait for her to come in before I would sit down.

Well, to make a long story short, we became "just friends." Cathy had another boyfriend and she would even tell me about their dates. But you know what? By becoming "just friends" we established a brother/sister relationship that served as a solid foundation between us. We spent a great amount of time talking and becoming closer friends. We had a great deal of fun together long before we became boyfriend and girlfriend.

I think that's why, after knowing each other for twelve years, we still like being together. We started off as friends rather than lovers. Far too often, though, people in a dating relationship do not work on establishing a friendship. That's why there can be so many hurt feelings and misunderstandings in some relationships.

## #3 Avoid Isolation

Another factor to consider in a dating relationship is to avoid isolating yourself. If you only spend time with your boyfriend or girlfriend and you have little time with your own friends, you probably have a poor relationship.

Often this imaginary scene happens in real life: Boy and girl meet. They like each other very much. They spend more time with each other. They come to enjoy each other's company so much that they begin to exclude their other friends. Finally they spend little or no time with anyone else. Their friends complain, but to no avail. Boy and girl become sexually involved. They break up. Both are feeling the heartbreak. Both feel like they've lost their other friends, too, and that they have no one to turn to in their loneliness.

In a positive dating relationship, even when people

are "going steady," they must maintain old friendships and spend time with other people. A positive relationship does not involve complete dependency; it involves a mutual love and respect that says, "I love you so much that I'm willing to share you with your friends."

## #5 Don't Stay Together Only for Security

One of the most difficult things to do in life is to break off a relationship, yet often it must be done. Most teenage relationships go on too long to be truly healthy. Then when they end there is much emotional trauma. Often one or both partners will attempt to restore the relationship. But there is nothing worse than trying to put back together something that should not be put back together. If you are hanging on to a relationship simply for the security it offers, muster up all your courage and break it off. The sooner you break up, the easier it will be.

Sometimes we don't know how to act around a person with whom we have ended a relationship. Try to continue to be friends. It might take time, but try to maintain a friendship. Perhaps it will eventually turn into a closer relationship. In order to do this, you'll have to stay away from gossiping or telling negative stories about your "ex." Try to put your differences aside and work at developing a brother/sister relationship.

## #7 Plan Fun and Enjoyable Dates

The average American date seems to consist of dinner, movie, and making out! I'm sure I'm exaggerating—but only a little! Since the purpose of dating is to become better friends, it's important to plan dates that will help

you get to know each other better. Many dates are boring because people do the same thing at the same time
at the same place. Sameness can cause even a good
relationship to go sour, so be creative with your dates.

In case you don't feel creative, here are more than
ninety creative and not-so-creative date suggestions.
I've compiled these over the years in brainstorming sessions with high schoolers and by reading a couple of
helpful books. Read through the list, think of other ideas
on your own, and be creative with your dating life!

## ACTIVE DATES/SPORTS

Ride a bike or bicycle-
  built-for-two
Visit a beach or lake
Ice skate
Shop
Play backgammon
Canoe
Go horseback riding
Try hiking or climbing
Dance
Play pinball or
  miniature golf
Water ski
Bowl
Try creative writing
  (poems, short stories)
Take up photography
Visit a batting cage
Play Ping-Pong
Play board games
  or card games
Plant a garden together
Wash your cars together

Take a walk
Roller skate
Play tennis
Learn racquetball
Sail
Go horseback riding
Fly kites
Fish
Ride a ferry
Attend a Bible study
Go for a drive
Snow ski
Jog
Get involved in handcrafts
  (Refinish an old piece of
  furniture! Experiment
  with ceramics!)
Take a fun class
  together (Conversa-
  tional French, photo-
  tography, watercolor
  painting)
Go on a scavenger hunt

Read a book aloud
  together
Do homework together
Collect something
  together
Play croquet

Go to the river for
  rafting or tubing
Play badminton
Build a treehouse
Ride motorcycles
Take an exercise
  class together

## FOOD

Go out to dinner—
  casual or fancy
Go home for lunch
  during the school day
Share a pizza and talk
Have a barbeque
Go on a picnic
Cook dinner for
  your parents

Take an ice cream
  break and talk
Kidnap the other person
  for breakfast
Cook dinner together
Bake cookies
Make homemade
  ice cream

## SPECTATOR

Attend a play
Go to the movies
Support school functions
Enjoy parties and friends
Go to a sports event
Visit a swap meet,
  an auction, or garage
  sales

Watch TV at someone's
  house
Go to a concert
Attend a Bible study
Watch hang gliders
Go to a public lecture
Hear a public speaker
Feed the ducks

## PLACES TO GO

The mountains
An interesting historical
  site
The circus

The beach
Museums
The zoo
The park and swing

The mountains in winter
  to play in the snow and
  build snowpeople
An observatory
The county fair

Church and youth
  group functions
The swap meet, an
  auction, or garage sales


**SERVE OTHERS**
Have a Bible study
Work at church together

Do volunteer work
  together


## Remember That Dating Is Preparation for Marriage

Not every person you date will be someone you would want to marry, but most of the people you date will become someone's marriage partner. That's why dating is good preparation for marriage. I think you should treat each date as a special date. In dating you can learn a lot about the type of person you would like to marry. As you date various types of people, you should get a better view of what you want in a mate.

At times it frightens me when two people who have dated only each other plan to get married. Most people need to experience a variety of relationships before they settle down for that one special life-long relationship. Listen to what a friend of mine told me recently: "I knew I loved Karen, but I never realized how much until one summer in college when we decided to date others. And, you know, that time really helped me see what it was I liked about Karen, and it only convinced me more that I was in love with her."

Another real benefit of dating is that you get a better idea of how you relate to the opposite sex in different situations. This can teach you some important things about yourself and about getting along with another person. And these lessons will help you be more sensitive and act more appropriately when you are ready to settle down and get married.

One last thought before we move on. Since each person you date is created by God and loved by our Lord, you should treat him or her with the same respect, dignity, and kindness that you want to receive from others. Remember, too, that many of the people you date will become someone else's spouse. And think about the fact that someone may be dating your future spouse right now.

## Avoid Getting Too Close Too Soon

My friend Mike Yaconelli recently gave me something to think about. He works with young people and really seems to understand what's happening among them today. He said, "Today it seems that too many kids take breaking up with a boyfriend or girlfriend way too hard. Their grief is almost as if they were married and going through a divorce." He then made this crushing statement: "I think it's because too many young people are having sex so soon after they meet that they are dealing with a deeper kind of intimacy than young people were even a few years ago."

You know what? Mike is right. Kids are becoming intimate so soon in their relationship that it is taking a terrible toll on their emotional health. Consider this scenario . . .

Tim and Susie like each other. In fact, they think they love each other. They hadn't meant to get so deeply involved physically, but they have. Call it curiosity, lust, sex drive, or just enjoying each other's touch. Whatever you call it, now they're in trouble. They've been intimate, but neither one is emotionally able to handle the deep commitment that goes with physical intimacy. The relationship begins to deteriorate until finally they break it off. It's too bad because they might have made a great couple. Instead, they must suffer the painful emotional consequences that come with breaking off physical intimacy.

If you have or would like to have a special relationship, move very, very slowly. That special friendship is worth the wait and the slower pace could possibly be one of the wisest decisions you will ever make. No one I've ever met who has waited to get physical in a relationship has ever regretted waiting. Think about that statement for a minute. I surely can't say the same about the number of my friends who didn't wait.

## Advice on Dating Non-Christians

Now for the big question. Should Christians date non-Christians? Every time I speak at a conference, every time I give a talk related to sex, and any time the subject of dating comes up, I am asked for my opinion on Christians dating non-Christians. Here it is.

Contrary to the belief of some people, all non-Christians are not interested in going to bed on the first date. All non-Christians are not pot smokers or heavy drinkers. I know many fine non-Christians. In fact, some of the kindest, gentlest, most talented people I know do not profess faith in the Lord Jesus Christ. I think it is a shame that well-meaning Christians give us advice that seems to say, "Stay away from those non-Christian pagans. They'll only pull you down!" It seems to me that Jesus said something about us Christians being the salt of the earth and the light of the world. Jesus spent time with sinners and helped them understand the real meaning of life. I think, then, that a Christian should be able to name some close non-Christian friends. I hope you are cultivating deep relationships with Christians and non-Christians alike.

I don't, however, believe in what some people call "missionary dating"—that is, dating a non-Christian in order to make him or her a Christian. Once in a great while this plan works but most often it leads to hurt, rejection, misunderstanding, and at times a real falling away from God. Although I believe we all need to have non-Christian friends, I'm afraid that when a Christian and non-Christian date it is like mixing apples and oranges.

Let me explain: There are no verses in the Bible that say "Thou shalt not date nonbelievers." There are, however, clear-cut guidelines that say we should not *marry* nonbelievers. Guess what? Dating leads to marriage.

I've seen too many relationships end in disaster when one person was a Christian and the other wasn't. I'm sure you've heard the horror stories also. Boy meets girl; they fall in love. Boy falls away from God because his new "god" is his girlfriend. Or boy meets girl and they fall in love. Boy and girl get married. Girl is a Christian, boy is not. Girl grows in one direction with one set of goals and standards while boy grows in the opposite direction with conflicting goals and standards. Boy and girl divorce with much heartbreak. I would imagine that when the apostle Paul advised against being yoked together with unbelievers (2 Cor. 6:14), he was writing out of his own experience of watching the heartache and confusion of "unequally yoked" (KJV) or "mismated" (RSV) people trying to have good marriages.

Scott Kirby gives what I think to be very sound advice in his book *Dating*: "Human beings are composed of body, soul and spirit. When a Christian marries a Non-Christian, the most they can have is two-thirds of a relationship."[1] I would simply add this: if you date non-Christians you are playing with fire. And not for the reason that they'll take you straight to hell. You are playing with fire because, while you may be very much alike, you are very different at the same time. Also, why settle for second best when you can have God's best in your life?

At this point, you might be objecting because I keep talking about marriage. You might even be saying, "There aren't any Christian guys or girls around here for me to date." I like Kirby's response: "If you usually date Non-Christians, then chances are you will marry a Non-Christian."[2] As I've said, the Bible is very clear when it comes to believers marrying non-Christians: "Do not be mismated with unbelievers. For what partnership have righteousness and iniquity? Or what fellowship has light with darkness?" (2 Cor. 6:14 RSV). Two people with two separate sets of goals and two separate "Lords" will have a very difficult time ever really coming together and developing a strong marriage.

My goal in this chapter has been to get you to think about what is best for you and your relationship with God. I caution you to think through your dating relationships seriously. It could mean the difference between a happy, fulfilled future and a future of disappointment and misery. When it comes to dating, don't settle for second best!

### Things to Think About

- What advice would you give a person who is ready to date but is not being asked out?
- Which suggestions on dating found in this chapter are most helpful for you? Why?
- Name two or three date ideas from the list in this

chapter that appeal to you and that cost little or nothing.
  • Can you add to the list of ideas for fun and enjoy-
able dates?
  • What is your opinion about dating non-Christians?
What facts and experiences is your opinion based on?

---

The *Handling Your Hormones* growth guide can
help you better understand Jim's views and your own
views of dating.

# CHAPTER 11

# Parties

When the phone rang, it was Jill's mother. (Jill was one of the sixteen-year-old girls in my youth group.) As I talked to her on the phone, Jill's mother seemed a little pushy and a little desperate. She said that recently Jill had "really changed for the worse." She was partying all the time, was losing interest in school, and had a bad attitude around the house. Her mother said that I had to help her wayward daughter and asked when I could meet with her.

It usually takes a while to get going in a counseling session. When a parent makes the appointment, the young person rarely wants to see me if he or she doesn't know me, and often he or she expects me to side with the parents—which I don't always do! But Jill and I hit it off almost immediately. She confided that she had been apprehensive about meeting me and I confided that I'd been apprehensive about meeting her, too!

After all the terrible things her mother had said, I couldn't believe that this was her daughter! Jill was open, honest, polite, and very friendly. This fact said to me that while she might have a bad attitude at home, she had a lot going for her. I could tell that Jill had as much potential as anyone I had recently met.

We met together a couple of times. Her story was like hundreds and hundreds of others. Yes, she was partying a little too much. Yes, she had experimented with drugs and alcohol. Yes, she was having more trouble in school, and it was also true that things weren't going so well at home. There was tension in the air—but it wasn't all from Jill. Her parents were experiencing a lot of stress at work and in their relationship with each other.

Despite this rather difficult situation, one thing in Jill's favor was that she said she was a Christian. In her words, "I'm not much of a Christian, but I do believe and I have a desire to grow in my faith." I believed her. I believed that she was sincere, and I asked one of our woman advisers to spend some time with her on a one-to-one basis. They went shopping, played a little tennis, and even started doing a weekly Bible study together.

It seemed like things were going much better for Jill. Then late one night I got a call from her. She had been to a party, she was very drunk, and she needed a ride home. My wife and I got out of bed and went to pick her up. By that time she had sobered up enough to talk sense, and she definitely needed to talk things out. She had not partied as much lately as she had before. But tonight's party had been important. Most of her friends had planned to attend, and a guy she really liked had kept asking if she was going to be there. He paid a lot of attention to her that night. They drank too much and Jill had blacked out. She was now sobbing in our car: "I think we went all the way, but I don't even remember." Jill was stunned, shocked at herself, and very depressed.

One day in my office a few months after what Jill called "the worst night in my life," we were talking about the need to discuss the topic of partying in our youth group. Jill and I came up with these five suggestions which we titled "Practical Guidelines for Partying." Take the time to read this list. Learn from Jill's experience! Don't wait to learn some of these lessons from personal heartbreak.

### If Partying Is a Weak Point in Your Life, Don't Go to Parties

Even if you enjoy going to parties, but find that you can't seem to control your actions as you would like, don't go. It's not worth the possible pain and hurt you might subject yourself to. Remember that we must live with our choices and their consequences, so choose—an act of your will!—not to go. Also, I think it is important to replace your old negative actions with new positive actions. If, for example, you have been a heavy partier and you want to stop, then don't just spend time watching TV and doing nothing. Replace the time you spent partying with other, more positive activities.

The key word here is "replace." It is much easier to overcome a bad habit or weakness in your life when you replace the negative experience with a positive one. My suggestion is that you actually write down on a piece of paper alternatives to partying that you would enjoy. Then when the temptation comes and you don't think you can handle the pressure, you can look at other possible options and choose one of those more positive experiences. A good list of possible replacements is in the preceding chapter on dating where I've listed nearly 100 date ideas.

### Host "Clean" Parties

It is not necessarily wrong to go to a party. All parties will not bring you down. To party really means to celebrate—and Christians have more to celebrate than anyone I know. Jill suggested that some of the Christians she knew could host what she called "clean" parties. The great thing about a party is spending time with people. Instead of going to parties where you have no control over what will take place, host parties that will be great fun and at the same time will keep you from getting into trouble.

## As a Christian, If You Go to Parties Invite the Lord Jesus to Go With You

Does that sound corny? It shouldn't. If you are a Christian, Jesus wants to be involved in everything you are involved in. If you actively invite Christ to attend a party with you, this awareness of Him will help you refrain from doing things that might disappoint both you and God. Also, you might be surprised to find that you have a better time than you've ever had!

## Choose Friends Who Will Help You Be the Best Person You Can Possibly Be

Jill had to take a serious look at the friends she was spending most of her time with. She finally decided that many of her problems stemmed from the type of people she had been hanging around with. At first she didn't think they were affecting her life-style, but when she really thought about it she realized that she had been compromising many of her beliefs because of peer pressure. Jill decided to choose close friends who would be a better influence on her and whose life-style would challenge her to live a more fulfilled life.

## Christians Do Not Live by the World's Standards

Jill asked me to add this guideline to the list. Her point is an important one, and perhaps Jesus said it best: "No one can serve two masters. Either he will hate the one and love the other, or he will be devoted to the one and despise the other" (Matt. 6:24 NIV). For most of us "wanting our cake and wanting to eat it, too" describes our desires. Most of us, if we are honest, want to live by the world's standards and also by God's standards. Sometimes we have to decide which is the very best standard to live by, and then go for it. Jill looked at and even experienced what the world could offer and what God could offer, and she chose God. She told me not long ago, "Not for one moment have I regretted my choice."

**Paul's Words to Us**

When God's standards seem rather abstract to us, that is when we need to turn to the Bible. I can think of several paragraphs written by Paul which set forth God's standards for us. These paragraphs really challenged me as a high school student, and they still challenge me today. I encourage you to take the time to read and study Colossians 3:1-17.

Arguing that since "you have been raised with Christ," Paul urges you to "set your hearts on things above, where Christ is seated at the right hand of God. Set your minds on things above, not on earthly things" (vv. 1-2 NIV). As he continues, Paul spares no words as he exhorts us to "put to death, therefore, whatever belongs to your earthly nature" and to "put on the new self, which is being renewed in knowledge in the image of its Creator" (vv. 5, 10 NIV). Paul then offers us some specific instructions:

> Therefore, as God's chosen people, holy and dearly loved, clothe yourselves with compassion, kindness, humility, gentleness and patience. Bear with each other and forgive whatever grievances you

may have against one another. Forgive as the Lord forgave you. And over all these virtues put on love, which binds them all together in perfect unity. (vv. 12-14 NIV)

Take time to read and study the passage in its entirety. Paul clearly defines the high standards we Christians should aim for in our daily life. These standards should apply to our behavior at parties as much as they should apply to any aspect of our life. Let me echo Paul as I close the chapter: choose friends and activities which honor God, don't invite temptation into your life, and trust God to be with you through whatever temptations might still arise.

---

## Things to Think About

• Do you think Christians should go to parties where there are drugs or drinking? Why or why not?

• What are the pros and cons of attending parties?

• What are some alternative ideas for things to do instead of partying?

• In Colossians 3:1 (quoted in this chapter), Paul tells Christians to "set your hearts on things above." What do you think that means?

---

# CHAPTER 12

# Drugs and Drinking

I'm no prude. In fact, many adults who read this book might think that I should be a little more prudish. But I'll be honest with you: Drugs and drinking scare me. Maybe it's because I've seen too many of the negative side effects of drinking in my own family. Maybe it's Steven, whom I met last year. At sixteen, his brain was fried from putting too many drugs into his body—and he had once had all the potential in the world for leading a happy and fulfilled life. Maybe it's Jill who got drunk and now isn't sure if she is a virgin or not. The list could go on; the stories only get worse, especially when you consider that most of the deaths in automobile accidents are caused by drunk drivers.

I'm also really frightened when it comes to what some people call the "mindbenders." I'm not going to tell you never to experiment with drugs and alcohol. The odds are that you've already tried one, if not both. I'm not going to tell you that every time you drink or take drugs horrible things will happen to you, because they won't. What I am going to tell you is this:

**Think Through Your Actions: Who's in Control?**

A person who is high is not in control of his or her

actions. Charlie Shedd wrote, "It is a good idea, where sex is involved to keep checking who's in control. Are you doing the thinking or is somebody else doing it for you? Do you really want to do this? Or are you doing it because somebody else is pressuring you?"[1] I've heard far too many stories about people who got high, couldn't control their actions and bingo, a pregnancy occurred—with all the lifelong effects that come with unwanted pregnancies.

### If You Drink, Don't Drive; If You Take Drugs, Don't Drive

I have a name for people who drink and drive: FOOLS.

Science has proven that even one beer can keep some people from being in control of their driving. A drunk driver (and I'm not necessarily talking about the type of drunk we see in the movies) is not only a dangerous weapon who may kill or maim himself or herself; a drunk driver has the definite ability to kill or maim innocent bystanders. If you drink or take drugs, don't drive.

Many people loved the move *Arthur*. It was the story of a happy drunk. To be honest, it depressed me greatly. Most drunks aren't *that* happy or *that* cute. Furthermore, most drunk drivers aren't as lucky as Arthur was when he drove through downtown New York City, barely missing other cars and pedestrians. *Arthur* was a make-believe story. If you want the real story, read your newspaper. Drunk-driving accidents happen every day, and most of the time they don't have happy endings.

### Alcoholism Is on the Rise

Fifteen percent of today's teenagers are alcoholics. Over

three million teenagers in the United States today are problem drinkers! They don't look or act like the stereotypical alcoholic. (Few people do!) They are addicted for life to something that has broken up more homes and ruined more lives than anything in the world. If you have even the slightest suspicion that you could possibly be an alcoholic, get help now. Don't wait until you hurt your family or ruin your life. Also, if you want to have an interesting experience, visit a local chapter of Alcoholics Anonymous (AA). You'll see very quickly that alcoholics are not happy people until they become recovered alcoholics; even then, many carry the scars of alcoholism for life.

The Bible says, "Don't drink too much wine, for many evils lie along that path; be filled instead with the Holy Spirit, and controlled by him" (Eph. 5:18 LB). I wish the Bible said, "Don't drink or take drugs; they will ruin your life!" But it doesn't. It simply says that we shouldn't get drunk (or high), but that we should be filled instead with the Holy Spirit. When you are high, you definitely cannot be allowing the Holy Spirit of God to work in your life.

I know a young person who chose not to drink when most of his friends and family drank. Some of his very close loved ones were alcoholics. I asked him once, "Why don't you drink?" I will never forget his answer: "I love the taste of some types of alcohol, and there is nothing better on a hot day than a cold glass of beer. *But I've decided I don't need it.* I'm not laying my trip on others, because I'm not convinced that everyone shouldn't drink; but let me tell you why I don't drink or take drugs. I could drink just one beer a week and see nothing wrong with it except that my alcoholic father would see that one beer and use it to justify his *case* of beer. I don't want to have a silent negative witness to my friends or family. And besides all that, I don't need to

drink or take drugs to be accepted. I'd rather be in control of my mind, spirit, and body at all times."

All I can add to this statement is, "Well said, my
friend; I can't think of anyone who wouldn't respect your
position."

## Drugs

I get nervous about any mood-altering substance. Too
many times I've seen my friends innocently get involved
with pot and end up with their brains "fried" on PCP or
acid (LSD). This doesn't mean that everyone who has
ever experimented with marijuana will end up in the
back of some alley with needlemarks up and down their
arms. However, anyone who becomes involved with any
mood-altering substance must carefully and logically
think through their actions.

Here's the straight scoop. Drugs work! They make
you feel good and they *will* get you high every single
time. Here's the problem. Because drugs alter your
mood, a person can easily become dependent on drugs.
The fact is that young people who take drugs at an early
age often quit coping with stress in a normal way and
become dependent on drugs to "make them feel better."
After a while people become preoccupied with getting
high because it is the only way they can function. And
most of the people who are preoccupied with getting
high are not the skid-row bums. They are the people
who have normal jobs and semi-normal families, yet if
you watch them over the years they bring a great deal of
tragedy into their own lives. What does all this mean? I
believe that there is a reason why they call this stuff
"dope" . . .

**Things to Think About**

• Why do you think some young people drink enough to get drunk?

• Are most teenagers able to control their drinking and drugs? Why or why not?

• Which philosophy of drinking do you feel closest to at this time of your life:

(_____) Never touch the stuff!

(_____) People can drink but not in excess.

(_____) It's a free country: people have the right to drink as much as they want.

• Without mentioning names, do you know of anyone who has had a negative experience with drugs or drinking? How has this affected your own thoughts about using drugs or alcohol?

• Do you think smoking marijuana is more harmful or less harmful than drinking alcohol? Why?

# CHAPTER 13

# Guilt and Forgiveness

Buffy is a seven-month-old puppy whose favorite meals are flowers, curtains, and tennis shoes. Every day my wife, Cathy, and I yell at Buffy and threaten her within an inch of her life. But it doesn't seem to help much. She just keeps chewing on anything and everything.

Here's a funny thing about Buffy, though. She almost seems to *know* when she has done something wrong. As soon as she has torn up my newest jogging shoes or eaten all the daisies Cathy put on the coffee table, she runs and hides under the kitchen table. And there she sits, looking as innocent as she can and trying to pretend nothing has happened.

But Cathy and I are wise to Buffy. We know that if that dog is under the kitchen table, it means that she has been up to no good. Sure enough, we don't have to look very hard to find evidence of Buffy's most recent mischief.

We human beings are a lot like Buffy. We do wrong things, and then we feel guilty for what we've done. We have a guilty conscience.

Dr. James Dobson tells about a poll that was taken among kids, asking, "What is conscience?" One six-year-old girl said a conscience is the spot inside that "burns if you're not good." A six-year-old boy said that he didn't know, but thought it had something to do with feeling bad when you "kicked girls or little dogs." And a nine-year-old explained it as a voice inside that says "no" when you want to do something like beat up your little brother.[1] One junior higher I know answered the same question by saying that a guilty conscience was "that sick feeling in the pit of your stomach when you realize you've just blown it."

Guilt, however, can be positive. Can you imagine what this world would be like if people didn't have consciences and didn't feel guilty when they did wrong? If human beings felt no guilt, the world probably wouldn't make it through another day. It would explode with sin.[2]

There are thousands and thousands of people in mental hospitals today because for one reason or another, they aren't able to deal with their feelings of guilt. I wish these people could understand that while guilt feelings have a necessary role in our lives, the great news of the gospel of Jesus Christ is that we can be *forgiven*. The guilt that drives us to seek forgiveness is then washed away. I believe that many people do not become Christians because they can't believe that the good news—the gospel—of Jesus Christ is true. They keep waiting for the catch to the story. But there is no catch. In Jesus Christ we can find forgiveness for our sins, past, present, and future! His death on the cross was the penalty He paid for your sins; the Resurrection from the tomb was His victory over sin and death and the gift of life for you. I know that idea is hard to understand, but nevertheless it is the truth. Consider the following story.

Sharon grew up in a basic middle-class American home. Her family seemed to fight more than the average family, but it was pretty much a normal family. They were not necessarily Christians, but in seventh grade Sharon went to church camp and decided to give her life to Jesus Christ. She became quite active in her church youth group, but peer pressure began to get to her and she experimented with light drugs and sex. One night when she was a tenth grader she got a little high and her twelfth-grade boyfriend convinced her to "go all the way." It was against her Christian principles, but she did it anyway. From that time on she seemed to slip down-hill emotionally. Life went on, but this one negative experience paralyzed her faith, her belief in herself, and her emotions.

I talked with her when she was in her early twenties. She still seemed paralyzed by guilt. After listening to her story for a long time, I asked her if she had ever asked Jesus Christ to forgive her for this past sin that kept haunting her. She replied, "Yes, almost every day since it happened in tenth grade." Eight years later she was still pleading for God's forgiveness.

I then asked her what I thought to be a simple ques-tion: "Do you believe God has forgiven you?"

Her answer gave me insight into her problem. She replied, "I really don't see how He could ever forgive me."

Even though Sharon was a Christian, she didn't understand the core of the gospel of Jesus Christ. We all do some pretty rotten things in life, but there is abso-lutely nothing that God will not forgive. God forgave our sins now and forever because of the sacrifice of Jesus on the cross.

Sharon needed to know—*really* know and believe in her innermost heart—that the very first time she asked for God's forgiveness, He had completely forgiven her. Her problem was that she would not accept His forgive-ness and she wouldn't forgive herself. Therefore, she carried around a load of *false* guilt that was ruining her life.

As you can see, God's ways are different from our ways. Humans tend to hold grudges and break off rela-tionships. God, however, always forgives. He always works to give His children new life. If you have not yet asked Jesus Christ to become part of your life, these next two paragraphs are for you.

The ultimate act of love was Jesus' death on the cross for you. The Bible says, "God demonstrates his own love for us in this: While we were still sinners, Christ died for us" (Rom. 5:8 NIV). I believe the most important decision in life is to acknowledge Christ's work on the cross and to invite Him to live within you. When you invite Christ to live in your life, He does a number of things immediately. I'll mention just a few: He forgives your sins, He dwells within you, He gives you eternal life, and He offers you an abundant life on earth.

If you have never asked Jesus Christ to come into your life, I urge you to do so right now. Here is a simple prayer. If you say it to God sincerely, your life will literally be transformed from the inside out. If you do say this prayer to God, then I urge you to get involved with Christians who will help you understand your new faith and will help you to grow as a new, forgiven believer. Here's the prayer:

"Almighty God, I love You. Thank You for the supreme sacrifice of love in Jesus Christ's death on the cross. I ask Jesus to come into my life and to forgive my sins. Thank You for setting me free. Amen."

Eventually Sharon did work through her guilt feelings and accepted the freedom and forgiveness Jesus offers. Today she is a happy, vibrant woman who understands that the forgiveness of Jesus Christ is a *free* gift given to all who ask. The Bible says, "If we confess our sins, he is faithful and just and will forgive us our sins and purify us from all unrighteousness" (1 John 1:9 NIV).

Perhaps you are a believer with a story similar to Sharon's. Now is the time to get rid of your guilt by asking Jesus Christ to forgive your sins. He is faithful to forgive you 100 percent of the time. When you ask, He forgives you, and you never have to feel guilty again.

One time someone asked me, "Aren't you afraid that kids will sin more if you tell them about God's complete forgiveness?" I replied, "Of course not! When a person really understands the unconditional love and forgiveness of Jesus Christ, the desire for obedience will be greater than the desire to sin." And I pray that you will believe this good news of Jesus Christ so that you will no longer be paralyzed by your guilt. The gift of forgiveness is yours for the asking. How can you pass up such an offer of love and total acceptance?

---

### Things to Think About

• Why is it so difficult to overcome our guilt feelings?

• Think of Sharon's inability to completely believe that God forgave her. What are some specific differences between real guilt and false guilt?

• What makes it difficult for you to accept God's forgiveness?

• What would you tell someone who has a guilty conscience?

---

Many of us struggle unnecessarily with guilt and an inability to accept the forgiveness God offers us. The *Handling Your Hormones* growth guide can help you learn more about the gracious and loving forgiveness which God promises you.

# CHAPTER 14

# Birth Control

Birth control is a tough issue. And some of you may even be wondering why, since I definitely oppose intercourse before marriage, I am including a chapter on birth control. By including it, am I teaching a person to "sin safely"? I don't think I am. Here's my view: If you choose to do wrong, for goodness' sake, use birth control to prevent any more heartache than you might already be causing by your actions. I like Charlie Shedd's advice. He calls it "Two Truths for Unmarried Teenagers About to Have Sex": "1. That boy who has intercourse without taking precautions is too irresponsible to deserve the name 'father'. 2. That girl who has intercourse without taking precautions is too irresponsible to deserve the name 'mother'."[1]

I'm frightened for the more than one million children a year born to American teenagers. I'm frightened for the American teenager who at age seventeen finds herself pregnant and feels ruined for life. Although I'm not advocating "easy" birth control, I think that for the sake of those one million babies and their mothers and fathers I need to discuss this important issue. I realize that many people will disapprove of my discussing birth control. When I share this with groups of parents, however, I would say that 95 percent agree with me and 5 percent disagree.

Here is a letter from a pastor who took the time to explain his reasons for believing that I shouldn't discuss birth control with students. I appreciate his openness and concern for following God's Word. I respect his sincere desire that we encourage obedience to God's commands. I feel, therefore, that it is important for you to read his opinion and then make up your own mind after you've considered both points of view.

Dear Jim:

I have gotten some feedback on the issue of talking to kids about birth control. I would imagine that the reaction of our people is the same that you would find in most other church groups. I've been chewing over the matter myself as I've talked to several people, and one thought that was expressed by the lady who spoke with you on the porch when you were leaving seems very appropriate. She said that there isn't anything "best" about God's second best. That term might imply that you only get the silver medal instead of the gold. Perhaps "cheap imitation" or "poor substitute" for God's very best would be a more appropriate phrase.

Some of the parents have asked their teens what their reaction would be to the parent discussing birth control with them. The consistent answer seems to be that the teen felt that the parent was giving indirect approval, or at least offering indirect acceptance, of sexual promiscuity.

I understand where you're coming from with your concern for not compounding sexual sin with pregnancy, but I am uneasy about parents instructing their child in how to sin safely. Pregnancy is certainly not the only consequence or scar that comes with being promiscuous, and the more I think about it the more I feel that the parents' efforts should be concentrated 100 percent on preventing the sin, not just on avoiding one of the consequences.

Signed,
A Brother in Christ

I really appreciate my friend's view, yet I still strongly believe that the best thing for me to do is to discuss birth control without condoning it. Someone needs to talk about it and I guess I'm the someone for now. And besides, when I talk about birth control in my "Handling Your Hormones" seminar, I feel that in general most of the kids are grateful for the information and understand that I'm not condoning sexual intercourse before marriage.

Before I discuss the various methods, let me say that no birth control method is completely safe. If you use a birth control method, please see a doctor and understand what you are using and why. If you are a Roman Catholic, realize that most of the methods I will describe are not acceptable to the Roman Catholic Church even for married couples. I would strongly suggest that you talk with a priest, nun, or religious instructor.

## The Pill

This little pill is usually made up of two hormones, estrogen and progesterone. With the pill, it is very unlikely that a woman will ovulate (release an egg for fertilization). The pill is very effective: only one in a hundred women per year get pregnant when using the pill correctly. There can, however, be negative side effects. These include possible water retention and weight gain, headaches, and breast tenderness. Other side effects can be irritability and moodiness. Some research centers are now seriously linking certain types of cancer and strokes to the pill. The pill is available by prescription only. You must see a physician to obtain the correct dosage. No one should "borrow" this or any medication from another person.

### The Condom (Rubber)

A condom is a thin rubber sheath that is placed over the penis to prevent the sperm from entering the vagina. If a condom is used properly, the pregnancy rate is three in one hundred. The condom will also help prevent the spread of venereal disease. One must make sure that the condom does not slip off during intercourse. If it does, the pregnancy rate increases greatly.

### Diaphragm

This is a thin rubber cap that is inserted into the vagina and fits over the cervix, the opening to the uterus. A diaphragm fails three out of one hundred times. Since the diaphragm must be the correct size for the individual, this form of birth control must be prescribed by a doctor for full effectiveness. Diaphragms are usually used in conjunction with spermicidal jelly.

### Contraceptive Foam

This spermicidal foam is inserted into the vagina by means of a plastic applicator. The chemicals in the foam kill the sperm as it enters the cervix. The failure rate is three in one hundred. If the foam is not applied properly, the rate goes much higher. Foam is available without a prescription.

**Natural Family Planning (Rhythm Method)**

This is the only "approved" manner of birth control for Roman Catholics. Here a woman must be constantly aware of her body and body temperature. At a certain time each month, she ovulates, releasing an egg from her ovary. The greatest chance for pregnancy is during ovulation. Often a woman can tell by a sudden drop in her temperature that she has ovulated. Of course, near this time of the month she must refrain from inter-course. If this monthly rhythm is watched carefully, the pregnancy rate is seven out of one hundred, but because of human error twenty out of one hundred is a more accurate number.

Many other forms of birth control exist, but they are more drastic and used less frequently than those meth-ods I've just described. In order for you to be informed, however, I will mention some of them.

**Sterilization**

Sterilization involves a vasectomy for men and a tubal ligation for women. In a vasectomy, the man's vas deferens (channels through which the sperm flows) are cut so that the sperm cannot mix with the semen. In a tubal ligation, the woman's Fallopian tubes are tied so that the egg and sperm cells cannot meet.

## Abortion

Abortion is a drastic means of birth control. Too many people who use this method have medical complications later such as scarring and damage to the female reproductive tracts, not to mention the emotional and psychological scarring that accompany an abortion. Sometimes infertility can result from an abortion.

## Intrauterine Device (IUD)

This is a small plastic device inserted into the uterus by a physician. This object stops the sperm before it can meet the egg. There is, however, a risk of infection, and some women experience heavier menstrual bleeding and cramping.

Still, there are other birth control methods which I have not mentioned. Some are not as popular and some are brand new. My strong suggestion to anyone who is sexually active is to talk with a responsible adult about all the various birth control methods, their possible side effects, and the responsibility that goes along with the choice to be sexually active.

Besides the various methods of birth control we've just looked at, there are many myths about birth control which you should also be aware of. Here are a few of them, along with the truth that contradicts the myth.

**Myth Number One**—You can't get pregnant the first time you have intercourse.
Whether it's your first or ninety-first experience doesn't make any difference. Any time you have intercourse, there is the possibility that you will become pregnant.

**Myth Number Two**—You can't get pregnant if you don't have an orgasm.
Whether or not you have an orgasm makes no difference at all. The sperm can still fertilize the egg and pregnancy will result if that happens.

**Myth Number Three**—You can't get pregnant if the penis is removed before ejaculation.
Before a man ejaculates, there is a lubricating fluid on the penis. This lubricating fluid may itself contain millions of sperm. Furthermore, it takes a lot of willpower to remove the penis from the vagina during intercourse before ejaculation occurs.

**Myth Number Four**—You can't get pregnant during your menstrual period.
Women have been known to become pregnant at any time during their cycles. Usually only one egg is released during a cycle. There can, however, be more than one egg released and an egg can also be released during a woman's period. Even though only one egg is released in most cases, the exact time of ovulation is difficult to determine, especially for young women because they tend to have irregular cycles.

**Myth Number Five**—Douching after sex will keep me from getting pregnant.
Sperm travel very quickly. Chances are that most of them have reached your uterus before you can sit up. Douches can also cause infection and upset the normal lining of the vagina.

Having outlined various methods of birth control and, I hope, having dispelled some of the myths surrounding birth control, I want to stress again that this discussion is *not* to be taken as my condoning premarital sex. I do, however, want to help you make a wise decision about sexual intercourse; I want to help educate you as to the risks and responsibilities involved; and I want to try to prevent future heartbreak that can come when sexual intercourse is entered into lightly.

## Things to Think About

- Do you believe birth control methods should be discussed with teenagers? Why or why not?
- Do most students have enough information about birth control?
- What do you think about Jim's statement: "If you choose to do wrong, for goodness' sake, use birth control to prevent any more heartache than you might already be causing by your actions"?
- What myth mentioned in this chapter do you think is most popular at your school?

# CHAPTER 15

# Options for the Pregnant

One of the reasons I've written this book is so that the subject of this chapter will never become a reality in your life. Unfortunately, the fact is that in the United States alone more than one million unwed girls and women become pregnant each year—and the number is increasing rapidly. Far too many times (perhaps most of the time) the people involved have not thought through the options until it is too late. Furthermore, often the pregnant girl must make some difficult decisions on her own because her partner has conveniently removed himself from the scene and is nowhere to be found.

To be honest, all the options for an unwed mother-to-be are lousy. All the options are complicated. All the options will cause a great deal of hurt and pain. Sometimes the difficulties are so great the girls simply won't admit that they are pregnant. They repress every thought about the subject until they actually believe that they are not pregnant—even after "the signs" begin to show. Too many people do not make decisions about their pregnancy because they simply wish it to go away. But it won't.

What can you do if you are pregnant? Here are some steps to take.

First of all, take a pregnancy test. Be 100 percent

sure that you are pregnant. If you have missed your peri-od or if you are even a little late, get checked as soon as possible. There is no sense second-guessing your body. The sooner you know for sure, the more time you will have to think through your options.

Today there are many easy ways to find out if you are pregnant. It takes approximately ten days after inter-course to know for sure, and there are methods being researched as of this writing that could possibly reveal a pregnancy as early as five days after conception. Early Pregnancy Tests (EPTs) are available without prescrip-tion at local drugstores, or you can go to your doctor, a hospital outpatient clinic, or a free clinic in your local area. If you use the Early Pregnancy Test and it indicates that you are pregnant, then you should immediately go to your doctor for confirmation and for instruction in prenatal care.

If you find out that you are pregnant, don't suffer alone. Share your situation with a person you trust. The best option is to sit down with one or both of your par-ents and have a heart-to-heart, open, and honest con-versation. Nine times out of ten, you'll find that you will receive more support than you expected. If you can't talk with your parents, find someone—a youth worker at church, a counselor at school, or a trusted adult friend—to confide in. You need all the positive support you can get.

Then take a very serious look at the options as rationally as possible. During stressful times, people often make emotional decisions that are simply wrong choices. These people mean well but fail to carefully consider all the options because of the emotional ten-sion in their lives.

At the age of twenty-five, Laura told me her own story of sadness and grief. When she was eighteen, she was homecoming queen, cheerleader, and president of her youth group. She became pregnant by an older man who immediately told her that she must get an abortion. Laura was confused, scared, and empty. Without telling family or friends, she went to another county in her state and had an abortion. It has been seven years and Laura has still not told her friends or family. Of course, her "boyfriend" is long gone. She told me that she really regretted having an abortion. She called it a "form of murder." Laura cried, "I may never be able to forgive myself." She never dreamed that she would be unmarried and pregnant. When she found herself in that predicament, she felt forced into aborting her baby. Now she lives to regret her actions.

I've heard too many similar stories. It always seems like it is the good, well-meaning people who make a mistake by never dealing with all the options. My wife and I sat with Janet and Bart. They were nineteen years old, intelligent, athletic, attractive, not married, and very (eight and a half months) pregnant. They were dealing with the difficult process of deciding whether to keep their baby or give the baby up for adoption. Neither choice was easy, and either one would change their lives forever. However, their social worker and my wife and I really sensed that even though they were confused, eventually Janet and Bart would make the decision which would be right for them. They were thinking rationally and looking at the options despite the intense emotional nature of the situation. Ultimately, they did give the baby up for adoption to two very special Christian parents who are making a wonderful home for this baby. I appreciated the maturity that Janet and Bart displayed as they took the time to work through the options before them.

Let's take a closer look at the options. The three possible options are abortion, adoption, and keeping the child. All three options have unique problems, but all three are options which you must consider.

## Abortion

Seldom in our nation's history has there been a more emotional issue than that of abortion. We all hear the various contradictory opinions. The pro-life people say that the living fetus within the mother is a human being with rights of its own—and the major right is the right to be born. These "right-to-life" people say that abortion is murder. Whew! These are strong words for the average young person to be dealing with—and the average older person as well!

On the other hand, the "freedom of choice" people say that women have the right to choose what they should do with their bodies. Most of these folks say that the fetus is really not human until a certain stage of pregnancy or until birth. Both sides play on our emotions. At many points, both sides make sense. Listening to all the views can be confusing.

I must be honest with you. I lean heavily toward the right-to-life option. Although the Bible doesn't say, "Thou shalt not abort," I feel that it does have something to say about the unborn fetus. Psalm 139:13-18 presents some important concepts for us to consider as we deal with this difficult issue. According to this beautiful psalm, God is actively involved in the development of the baby in the mother's womb. As the psalmist begins this passage, he writes, "For you created my inmost being; you knit me together in my mother's womb" (v. 13 NIV). According to this Old Testament poet and probably to any woman who has ever carried a child, a fetus seems to be unquestionably a human being created and loved by our Maker.

I have friends who have had abortions, though. I've

counseled people after abortions. Believe me when I tell you that the abortion experience is incredibly hard on the girl or woman who goes through it. I definitely do not love or respect these people any less. And I believe that God doesn't love them any less either. Many people, however, seem to have trouble living with themselves after an abortion. Guilt, hurt, emptiness, and regret may fill the person's being in such a way that she is unable to cope with the emotions or the memories. Whatever you do or whatever you decide, count the cost. There is usually a psychological, spiritual, and emotional price to pay for the decision to abort.

If you choose to have an abortion, make sure that you get the very best medical and counseling advice ahead of time. By all means, do not go to a second-rate facility to have an abortion. Perhaps most important of all, see a qualified counselor who can help you deal with the issues involved with an abortion. Often when a young girl realizes she is pregnant, she will be in such a confused and emotional state that she will simply follow the advice of the people closest to her. She will feel forced into making a decision that she might eventually regret. Remember that the person who is pregnant must make the ultimate decision about her body. Take your time and look at all the issues.

## Adoption

Although adoption is not as popular as it used to be, it is definitely still an important option. Adoption can be a very positive alternative to abortion or keeping the baby. It can be a very positive experience for the birth parents, the child, and the adoptive parents.

At seventeen, Anne felt that she was too young to raise the child she was carrying. Her boyfriend was sticking beside her through the pregnancy, but he wasn't ready to settle down. With the help of a counselor, Anne carefully considered the options and decided to give up her baby for adoption. The adoptive parents were a young couple in their late twenties. They had been married for five years and had been told that they would never be able to have children of their own. They desperately wanted to raise children and give them a home. A medical doctor made the arrangements for Anne's baby to be adopted by this couple. Anne was reassured that her child would be given to very special people who would provide a warm, loving home for the baby. When she delivered, Anne allowed the adoptive parents to take the baby home from the hospital. Later Anne wrote a letter to the new parents and mailed it to her doctor who sent it on to the couple. This is what she wrote:

Dear Parents of the Little Baby:
    I want you to know that I pray for your—I mean "our"—child daily. As I look back on the decision to give up my baby for adoption, it was the most difficult decision I've ever made.
    But I want you to know, too, that it was also the wisest decision and I know the best decision for the baby. I hope you'll tell the baby when he grows up that I love him and will always love him. Help him understand that I gave him up because I wanted the best for him.
    Even though I've never met you and probably never will, I'm grateful to God for the love you have for "our" child.
                    With all my love,
                    Unsigned

    Should you decide to give up your baby for adoption, make sure that you go through a respectable agency whose number one desire is to give your baby the finest home possible. Make sure that the agency or lawyer or whoever handles the adoption does a thorough home study of the adoptive family. One of the biggest issues in the mind of every birth parent is whether the baby will live in a happy, secure home that is filled with love and support. When a person is confident that the baby will be in such a home, it is easier to give up the baby to adoptive parents.

**Keeping the Baby**

An option that seems to be gaining in popularity among young people is keeping the baby. Today more than ever before we see young girls deciding against abortion or adoption; instead they are raising their babies themselves. Here I have mixed emotions. If a young person can handle the responsibility of child raising, she should consider very strongly keeping the baby. Most young people, however, have a terribly difficult time managing their own problems let alone a baby's constant pleas for love and attention. I'm amazed at the amount of child abuse that consequently occurs among teenage parents. The statistics are frightening.

If you are pregnant and are trying to make a decision about keeping the baby, ask yourself questions like these: What is the best for the baby? Will I get married to the father? Am I emotionally stable enough to handle the constant demands of child raising? Also, make sure that you get help from a counselor. I know a number of great kids who were born to teenage parents and who have turned out fine. I also know some young people who have been raised by teenage parents and who have had real emotional struggles due to being raised in a difficult home situation. Your decision to keep the child must be a personal decision, but get the advice and help of people who sincerely love you and want the best for you and the baby.

Charlie Shedd wrote a great book on sex entitled *The Stork Is Dead*. Written in 1968, it still offers what seems to be timeless insight. He quotes, for instance, a letter written to him by a young girl on what it's like to be married at seventeen. It's worth reprinting here.


Jimmy and I couldn't wait so now we are married. Big deal!

Let me tell you what it is like to be married at 17. It is like living in this dump on the third floor up and your only window looks out on somebody else's third floor dump.

It is like coming home at night so tired you feel like you're dead from standing all day at your checker's job. But you don't dare sit down because you might never get up again and there are so many things to do like cooking and washing and dusting and ironing. So you go through the motions and you hate your job and you ask yourself, "Why don't I quit?" and you already know why. It's because there are grocery bills and drug bills and rent bills and doctor bills, and Jimmy's crummy little check from the lumber yard won't cover them, that's why!

Then you try to play with the baby until Jimmy comes home. Only sometimes you don't feel like playing with her. But even if you do, you get this awful feeling that you are only doing it because you feel guilty. She is so beautiful, and you know it isn't fair for her to be in that old lady's nursery all day long. Then you wash diapers and mix formula and you hate it, and you wonder how long it will be till she can tell how you feel, and wouldn't it be awful if she could tell already?

Then Jimmy doesn't come home, and you know it's because he is out with the boys doing the things he didn't get to do because you had to get married. So, finally you go to bed and cry yourself to sleep telling yourself that it really is better when he doesn't come because sometimes he says the cruelest things. Then you ask yourself "Why does he hate me so?" And you know it is because he feels trapped, and he doesn't love you anymore, like he said he would.

Then he comes home and he wakes you up, and he starts saying all the nice things he said before you got married. But you know it is only because he wants something, and yet you want to believe that maybe it is the old Jimmy again. So you give in, only when he gets what he wants, he turns away and you know he was only using you once more. So you try to sleep but you can't. This time, you cry silently because you don't want to admit that you care.

You lie there and think. You think about your parents and your brothers and the way they teased you. You think about your backyard and the swing and the tree house and all the things you had when you were little. You think about the good meals your mother cooked and how she tried to talk to you, but you were so sure she had forgotten what it was like to be in love.

Then you think about your girlfriends and the fun they must be having at the prom. You think about the college you planned to go to, and you wonder who will get the scholarship they promised you. You wonder who you would have dated in college and who you might have married and what kind of a job would he have had?

Suddenly you want to talk, so you reach over and touch Jimmy. But he is far away and he pushes you aside, so now you can cry yourself to sleep for real.

If you ever meet any girls like me who think they are just too smart to listen to anyone, I hope you'll tell them that this is what it is like to be married at seventeen.[1]

As this story and the entire chapter have pointed out, the decision facing unwed teenage mothers is not an easy one. If you find yourself in this situation, it is important that you think through the options as carefully and as unemotionally as possible. It is also important that you really try to listen to the advice of those people who care about you and whom you can trust. Also, lean on God for His strength in this difficult time, for His answers to your prayers for guidance, and for the peace which He offers to His children.

---

**Things to Think About**

• What is your opinion of each of the three options we've discussed—of abortion, adoption, and keeping the baby?

• List the pros and cons of each option.

• Why do you think some people simply deny that they are pregnant?

• Who do you know who would be helpful to talk to about subjects like this? Consider, for example, a minister, a school counselor, or an adult friend.

---

Use the *Handling Your Hormones* growth guide in conjunction with this chapter. Better define for yourself your own ideas abut the options for an unwed teenage mother-to-be.

CHAPTER 16

# Masturbation

Even the sound of the word "masturbation" causes strange reactions in most
people. Masturbation is, however, an experience which
most people have had, yet seldom does anyone talk
about it. And when so-called experts discuss or write
about the subject, they can't seem to agree on whether it
is right or wrong.

Some people are uncertain about what masturbation actually is. Technically, masturbation is called
"autoeroticism." "Auto" means "self" and "erotocism"
means "sexual stimulation." Put the words together and
you have "self sexual stimulation." Masturbation is the
fondling or stroking of one's own sexual organs to produce a pleasant sexual sensation. Masturbation is usually the first sexual behavior for both males and females.
Often you'll find little children handling their genitals
and exploring their bodies, but even then their parents
may discourage this behavior.

About nine years ago I was a counselor at a Christian
camp. I was working with eight high school guys. Somehow in our morning Bible study time the subject of
masturbation came up. I discussed it openly and honestly with these guys. Before lunch the word was out:
"Jim doesn't think all masturbation is sinful!" Before
lunch was over the man in charge of the camp had

pulled me aside to ask just what we were talking about during the Bible study hour. I told him the same thing that I told the guys in my cabin and that I am telling you. Incidentally, before that camp was over, at least twenty high schoolers asked if they could talk with me privately about their problem. This says to me that it is time we become more open about this important subject and help people deal with their "problem" in an intelligent manner.

Almost all people have had a masturbation experience by the time they reach eighteen years of age. A person is not abnormal if he or she has never had the experience and a person is not abnormal if he or she has had it. Statistics tell us that in the last twenty-five years many more girls have masturbated than ever before. I've read statistics that say between 50 and 80 percent of all girls have had a masturbation experience. I've heard it said that 92 percent of all males have had the experience and the other 8 percent are liars. In other words, almost all males have had the experience. I tell you these statistics because far too many people believe that they are among just a few people in the world masturbating. They are completely wrong.

"Okay, Jim, but let's get to the point: is masturbation wrong? Is it a sin?" If I must be pinned down, I believe that not all masturbation is necessarily sinful. However, you must make up your own mind. You must intelligently work through the decision. And I would suggest that you turn to God for help. Let me give you two opposing viewpoints from two outstanding Christian people to help you arrive at your decision.

First, in his book *This Is Loving?*, David Wilkerson says, "Masturbation is not a gift of God for release of sex drives. Masturbation is not moral behavior and is not condoned in the Scriptures . . . . Masturbation is not harmless fun."[1] On the other hand, Charlie Shedd, a very respected Christian authority on sex and dating, does call masturbation a "gift of God." He claims that masturbation "can be a positive factor in your total development" and goes on to say that "teenage masturbation is preferable to teenage intercourse. It is better to come home hot and bothered than satisfied and worried."[2]

My own view is somewhere in between these two extremes. Masturbation is practically universal. It isn't the gross sin some people think it is, yet at times it can have a negative side to it.

Specifically, uncontrolled masturbation can be very negative. Psychologists call this type of behavior "obsessive-compulsive." This means that a person can become so consumed with masturbation that it literally takes over his or her mind and actions. One young man confided to me that he figured he masturbated ten to fifteen times a week and that this one experience had literally taken over his mind. He had tremendous guilt feelings, was drawing more and more into himself, and was afraid to be with people. His obsessive-compulsive behavior was destroying his self-image, his relationship with God, and his relationships with other people. We had to help him work through his negative habit and change his behavior.

Another negative effect is uncontrolled fantasy. Jesus loves us unconditionally and yet He calls us to high standards. When discussing the question of lust, for instance, Jesus said, "You have heard that it was said, 'Do not commit adultery'. But I tell you that anyone who looks at a woman lustfully has already committed adultery with her in his heart. If your right eye causes you to sin, gouge it out and throw it away. It is better for you to lose one part of your body than for your whole body to be thrown to hell" (Matt. 5:27-28 NIV). When masturbation leads to uncontrolled fantasy, God calls it a sin.

Often people who struggle with an overactive fantasy life are reading pornographic literature, watching X-rated movies, and constantly placing themselves in a position to be aroused by sexually stimulating material. I am convinced that those who have a problem with their fantasies should stay away from any pornographic material. Their fantasy problem, even if it does not disappear completely, will definitely be easier to control.

One more thing. If you are filled with negative guilt feelings and a real sense of insecurity, don't suffer in silence. Even though it is a difficult subject to discuss, share your feelings and questions with someone you can trust. Your feelings might be well-founded, but on the other hand, they might simply be false guilt.

## The Not-So-Negative Factors

I'm afraid that too many times well-meaning parents, friends, teachers, and ministers have added coals to the fire when the tell kids, "If you do it, you will become sterile, blind, mentally ill, or homosexual." There is no truth whatsoever in those suggestions. Whatever else can be said about masturbation, most doctors, scientists, psychologists, and ministers now agree that it will not harm you biologically. Let me repeat an earlier statement: If you've had the experience you are normal; if you haven't, you are also normal.

Dr. Herbert J. Miles, in his excellent little book *Sexual Understanding Before Marriage*, makes a case for a limited program of masturbation for young men who, biologically, are at the peak of their sexual drive. For young men at this point of their lives, "we feel that a rigid condemnation of all masturbation as being sinful is rather arbitrary, unrealistic and out of harmony with the creative plan of God."[3] Dr. Miles goes on to emphasize the necessity for sexual self-control before marriage. He argues that a young man "must never violate another person to meet his sexual needs. He must lean on nocturnal emission (wet-dreams) and sublimation and he may when needed supplement them with a temporary, limited program of masturbation."[4]

One statistic to consider is the positive trend in today's American society toward getting married at a later age. I say it is a positive trend because most teenage marriages do not make it. But because people are waiting longer, their sexual adrenalin must also wait longer. It seems to me that a limited amount of masturbation will relieve the sexual tension and not do the harm that people once thought it would. My own feeling is that we've made too big an issue of this subject. We've produced too much guilt and we have seldom mentioned the subject except in a negative way.

To be perfectly honest, as a Christian, I wish the Bible gave us a clear-cut answer. It does not. The Bible simply does not discuss this issue. As much as I would like to give you *The Answer*, I cannot. There isn't one. Here is a subject that you will have to work through alone or with the help of someone you trust. The book of James gives some solid advice, though: "If any of you lacks wisdom, he should ask God, who gives generously to all without finding fault, and it will be given to him" (James 1:5 NIV). Let God help you make a decision that is glorifying to Him. Remember, He created you—and your sexual identity!

---

**Things to Think About**
• Why do you think people are so silent about masturbation?

• Three views are given about masturbation: Dr. Miles's, Dr. Shedd's, and David Wilkerson's. Of these three views, do you think any one of them is more in line with the general principles of Scripture than the others?

• Jim mentioned the words "uncontrolled fantasy." How can that be a negative factor?

• Do you believe Jim was right or wrong to discuss the topic of masturbation with the high school guys at the camp? Do you feel adults should talk openly with teenagers about sex and related matters?

# CHAPTER 17

# Venereal Disease

When it comes to the subject of vene-real disease, most of us try to forget that it even exists. ("Venereal" refers to something related to or transmitted by sexual intercourse. "Venereal disease" is any one of several diseases contracted mainly through sexual intercourse.) Each year, however, there are over three million cases of venereal disease in the United States. In fact, gonorrhea now ranks second only to the common cold among communicable diseases. And because more people are having casual sex these days, the spread of "sexually transmitted diseases" is at an epidemic level, according to the American Medical Association. I believe, therefore, that it is important for every person, sexually active or not, to understand venereal disease, the symptoms, the consequences, and the treatments.

## Gonorrhea

Gonorrhea is the most common of venereal diseases. Basically, the only way to get the disease is through sexual contact. One dangerous feature of gonorrhea has earned it the name the "silent disease": sometimes there are no major symptoms when a person has contracted it. In fact, a person may go for years without knowing that he or she has the disease. In the meantime, serious physical damage may occur.

Usually, however, there are symptoms. Two to seven days after contact with someone who has gonorrhea, a woman might have a vaginal discharge, maybe mild pain upon urination, and perhaps an abnormal menstrual period. A man's symptoms usually include a painful, burning sensation when he urinates and an uncomfortable discharge from the penis.

There is a cure for gonorrhea. Penicillin can cure the disease if it is found in the first stages. Without treatment, however, a person can become sterile (unable to produce children) because of damage to the sperm ducts or the Fallopian tubes. Gonorrhea has also been known to cause arthritis, meningitis, and heart disease. Another very sad effect of gonorrhea is that it can cause blindness in an innocent baby at birth. These are not scare tactics about V.D.—these are medical facts!

### Syphilis

Syphilis is a dangerous disease. Among communicable diseases, it is a major killer. If not treated in the first or second stages, syphilis can cause infections which will affect the heart, the brain, and the spinal cord, causing serious deterioration of the body.

There are basically three stages of syphilis. The first symptom usually appears between ten and ninety days after contact. Usually a painless canker sore will appear on the penis or in or near the vagina. The canker sore will disappear after a few weeks. The second stage, which usually occurs between two and six months after contact, manifests itself as a rash all over the body with possibly a few sores on the sex organs. Tragically, by the time the disease reaches the third stage (often fifteen to twenty-five years after it has been contracted), it is very difficult to treat. It can invade the nervous system, cause paralysis, and result in insanity. Blindness, swollen joints, and crippling can also come in the advanced stages of syphilis.

## Genital Herpes

Today the most talked about form of venereal disease is herpes simplex II. Perhaps you have read about the outbreak of herpes in our country. Genital herpes is causing some sexually active people to at least be more selective about their partners because at this time there is no known cure for herpes.

Within three weeks of sexual contact with a partner infected by herpes, a person will develop blisters around the genitals. There may be painful urination, fatigue, and swelling in the groin area. The blisters will pop after a few days, leaving a discharge, and then the symptoms will go away. This does not mean that the symptoms won't come back. Periodically the blisters and some of the other signs will appear, often without pain. The medical profession is desperately trying to find a cure, but so far all they have is a treatment that may reduce pain and help prevent secondary infection.

As you can see, and contrary to what you may have heard, venereal disease is very serious business. If you have even the slightest symptoms of a venereal disease, go immediately to a physician. Yes, it is embarrassing, but these diseases cannot be "wished" away. Today in the United States, for every reported case of venereal disease there are thought to be two or three unreported cases. Perhaps some of those people do not recognize the signs, but many of them are simply afraid to report their symptoms. They wish and hope the signs will go away and thus risk suffering major physical consequences.

In today's society, it is very easy to be sexually promiscuous. There are people in such desperate need of attention that they will go from one bed partner to another. With venereal diseases at epidemic levels, these people are playing with fire that literally can be deadly.

A young married man named Jim talked with a nurse named Arvis Olsen and asked for the latest information on cures for herpes II. Mrs. Olsen recorded this conversation in her excellent book *Sexuality: Guidelines for Teenagers*. Read Jim's comments carefully and look at the negative consequences he and his wife suffered.

Jim came to me and asked for the latest information on cures for Herpes II. "I got this pesky disease during college and have never been able to get rid of it. Every few months I get blisters, then they disappear, only to return again later. I wasn't too worried about it until my wife's last visit to her doctor for her yearly checkup. He says she has to have a repeat on her Pap smear because the first test showed cell changes on her cervix. He told her that cervical cancers could be caused by the Herpes virus, and he also told her she would be wise not to have any more children. We have only one child, Nurse, and I'm scared to death—let me add that all this has not done a lot for our marriage. If only I had known the consequences of the 'fooling around' I did when I was nineteen! Marge and I could have the happiest marriage in the world, except . . . Those moments of pleasure were foolish, and the payment is unrelenting."[1]

Most people do not want to think about venereal disease, and they especially do not want to think that it could happen to them. Yet statistics tell us that venereal disease continues to exist on an epidemic level. It won't go away just because people wish it to. Furthermore, sexually active young people today need to know the facts about venereal disease because the odds are in favor of a sexually active young person contracting this disease. One young friend of mine who contracted gonorrhea said to me, "It never entered my mind that I would get the disease. I thought it only happened to bad people. I don't think the sexual contact was worth the pain or humiliation." Remember, venereal disease is no respecter of persons.

---

### Things to Think About

- Do you feel that students are informed enough about the venereal diseases?
- Do kids at school ever talk about venereal disease?
- What is your opinion of "casual sex"?
- Do you think that because there is no cure for genital herpes some people will refrain from casual sex?

---

# CHAPTER 18

# Homosexuality

When Mike came into our youth group a number of years ago, the group loved and accepted him immediately. It was easy to like him: he was fun-loving, outgoing, athletic, and intelligent, and he had a real desire to grow in his new-found Christian faith. I wonder how the kids would have accepted him if they had known, as I did, that he was homosexual. I would cringe at times when some of the other kids in the group would tell "queer" jokes or would pretend to act feminine with a limp wrist in the air to get laughs. I would often catch myself stealing a quick glance at Mike. He never let on around the guys that it bothered him, but he sure let me know. We would talk and talk about his feelings about being gay and being Christian—which brings up a good question. Can a person be a homosexual and a Christian at the same time? I believe that the answer is a definite yes. Although the Bible calls the homosexual act a sin, in the same passage it lists envy, deceit, and gossip as equally sinful as the homosexual act. (See Rom. 1:26-32.)

Any discussion of homosexuality is very complicated. But let's begin with the fact that all homosexuals are loved by God. He might not be pleased with the act of homosexuality, but He definitely loves the homosexual. In fact, all Christians should love homosexuals unconditionally not for what they do or don't do, but for who they are. They are loved by our Lord just as much as heterosexuals are.

Who is the homosexual? Many young people are confused about this subject, and one reason is that they may have had one homosexual experience and they think they might be gay. Many, perhaps most, young people do have what one might call a homosexual experience. Children, for instance, are very curious and "play doctor" or engage in other types of experimentation. If this has happened to you, it does not mean that you are a homosexual. It means that you, like millions of others before you, have had a normal childhood experience. Even if you as a teenager have had a few homosexual experiences, this does not mean that you are gay. A homosexual person is a person who has had continued sexual activity with others of the same sex and/or is primarily attracted to those of the same sex. The person attracted to both sexes is called a bisexual.

What causes homosexuality? All the information is not in yet. Some experts believe that homosexuality is genetic in origin. Others suggest that it comes from a hormone imbalance. Some researchers feel very strongly that homosexuality is caused by a negative home environment, perhaps an overly dominant mother or a poor role model for a father. I guess the best answer is that no one really knows exactly what causes homosexuality, and I'm sure that the answer is very complicated. In fact, the answer is probably a combination of some or all of the factors I've mentioned.

One thing is very clear. If you are a homosexual, it is not necessarily your fault, but I like what Tim Stafford of *Campus Life* says. He writes, "The condition has been given to you. You're accountable for how you respond."[1] Many homosexuals blame other forces for their behavior. I understand their logic and I hurt for them, but I agree with Stafford. The homosexual has the final responsibility for his or her sexual behavior. I have met people who will probably have a homosexual tendency all of their lives. They may be like alcoholics—once an alcoholic, always an alcoholic, even if they never indulge. Many Christians who do have a tendency toward homosexuality have, however, chosen to refrain from homosexual actions. The sin is in the actions, not the "tendency."

Most heterosexuals do not understand what it is like to be a homosexual. They view with repugnance the actions of practicing homosexuals. As Christians, however, we must take the biblical stance of unconditional love for our brothers and sisters. I believe, too, that it is important for us to understand this problem because within our culture we will increasingly come into contact with people confused about their sexuality.

If you feel you might be a homosexual, seek counsel. The longer you wait, the harder it is to understand your sexual identity. Meet with a counselor you trust and share with him or her your inner thoughts. You are not a freak! Many people share your confusion. Another piece of advice. When you are confused and hurting, don't drink or take dope. Many sexually confused people go to the bottle, pills, or marijuana to "overcome the problem." This "solution" doesn't work; in fact, it usually causes more problems.

Having encouraged you to seek counseling, I want to say one other important thing. If you want to change, I believe that you can. First, it takes a strong desire to change. Second, you need God's supernatural power in your life to give you the extra support you need. Get involved in church, read the Bible, and pray daily. Third, find a wise counselor who will listen to you, care about you, and hold you accountable to your resolution to change. It is also very important to leave your friends who have had a negative influence on you and find a new set of friends who will be positive influences. Find friends who enjoy life and challenge you to be all that God desires you to be. I strongly recommend that you get involved with Christian friends and become active in a church.

Let me close with a story of hope. Carl was a sixteen-year-old who, though very shy, was a consistent participant in my youth group. One day while on a camping trip, he confided to me that he thought he was gay. He had been involved in various "gay" relationships for two years, yet he felt very unfulfilled and guilt-ridden. He wanted to change but felt chained to his gay life-style. He asked if I could help.

Since Carl had a strong desire to change, I affirmed his desire and got him involved in some good counseling. I went with him to his first appointment for support. Although the counseling was somewhat painful for Carl, it was also life-changing. He moved to another area of our state but continued in counseling and became very active in his new church. Today Carl is married and has a little child. He says, "God used the counseling, the strong support from Christian friends, and my church to free me from my bondage."

---

**Things to Think About**

- Do you believe it is a sin to be homosexual? Why or why not?
- What would you do if one of your friends confided in you that he or she is a homosexual?
- Can you be a Christian and a homosexual?
- Do you think it is okay to make fun of homosexuals? Why or why not?

---

# CHAPTER 19

# Bad Experiences

This is a very difficult chapter to write. I struggle about including it. It seems, however, that no one today is exempt from the harsh reality that tragic experiences happen to both good and bad people. If you or a friend of yours has faced some of the difficult experiences mentioned in this chapter, seek outside help. This chapter does not provide all-inclusive information. It is written as an overview and as a catalyst for action.

## Rape

Rape is perhaps the ultimate outrage. Rape is one of the most horrible crimes committed against a person of the opposite sex. Rape is most often inflicted *not* as a sexual crime but as a violent crime. Most rapists are not so much interested in sexual pleasure as in hurting and frightening the victim. There is usually a great deal of anger, aggression, and hatred within the psychological makeup of the rapist. Most victims of rapes are women and girls, although in the last few years there has been an increase in the number of homosexual rapes of men and boys. In this chapter, for convenience, I will refer to rape victims as women.

A person who has been raped should immediately go to a nearby hospital or rape crisis center. Here she will be checked for injuries. The doctor should also check for and collect evidence of the rape. The victim should not wash up before going to the hospital or center. You'll find that almost all the people, from doctors and nurses to police officers, are very caring individuals who will compassionately help the rape victim through her initial shock and pain. A rape victim should not go through this process alone. She should get the best medical treatment available along with some professional counseling. Many trained individuals can and will make recovery from this painful experience a little easier.

Even better than coping with rape is preventing it. The very best protection is to stay away from potentially dangerous situations. Too many people have not thought through their actions and have lived to regret it. Here are a few suggestions to help prevent a rape. I encourage you to get in touch with your local rape prevention or crisis center for even more information.

1. Never hitchhike. You're asking for trouble.

2. Don't walk or jog alone at night. This can be very dangerous.

3. Carry a whistle. Put the whistle on your key chain and keep it in your hand when you are alone.

4. Don't go out alone with a person you don't know. Too many people have been "picked up" at a dance, amusement park, or other public place without realizing that they were "picked up" by a rapist.

5. Don't flirt with someone you don't know. You could be flirting with a rapist.

**Incest**

Incest is having sexual relations with a member of your

own family, and sadly incest is far more common than most people imagine. The most common form of incest is a father-daughter relationship, but there are many cases reported each year of sexual relations between mother and son or brother and sister as well as between other relatives.

Incest is a very serious and sensitive subject because it deals with family members, but there is no such thing as a positive experience involving incest. An incestuous relationship must be stopped. If you or someone you know has been involved with incest, do not keep it to yourself. Report it to a proper authority immediately. A good place to start would be a minister, social worker, counselor, or police officer. The victim of incest will need help and so will the aggressor. Sometimes victims of incest believe that the experience is their own fault. Such faulty thought patterns produce extreme but completely unnecessary guilt and self-blame. The victim of incest is not at fault and should not take on the blame for someone else's sickness. Furthermore, no one is doing the aggressor a favor by keeping quiet about the problem.

At age sixteen, Linda confided in me that she had been forced into an incestuous relationship with her father from the time she was seven until she was thirteen. I never would have guessed her problem in a million years. She appeared on the outside to have it all together, but on the inside she lived with tremendous amounts of hurt, anger, bitterness, and guilt. By the time she saw me, she was a volcano ready to explode at any minute.

Here are the steps I went through with Linda. First, as her youth pastor, it was important for me to be a support and encouragement to her. She needed someone to lean on, so my wife and I both became good listeners for her. Second, we felt she needed extensive counseling and so we referred her to an experienced psychologist and trusted friend. We let him deal with the major psychological trauma and we continued as supportive friends and pastors. At the right time, the psychologist made contact with her father and found that he was open to getting counseling. Over the next two years, we watched a broken relationship mend. There are still scars and at times there is resentment, but Linda has blossomed into a beautiful young woman both inside and outside. On her wedding day, she was able to allow her father to walk her down the aisle.

Having worked through a difficult situation, Linda now says she would not have been able to do it without God's help and the healing and loving support of friends. Somehow she was able to understand God's love and forgiveness for herself and for her father. It wasn't easy, and some people are not as fortunate as Linda. They may never be able to forgive their aggressor. In situations involving incest, no one should expect instant forgiveness or the instant healing of broken relationships. It may require a long time for the victim to reach the point of forgiving the aggressor. Still, I believe all people who have experienced the devastation of incest should seek help. There *is* hope—just ask Linda.

## Pornography

Far too often, pornography fills the void caused by the lack of sex education at home, church, or school. Almost all young people have seen or read some form of pornography. Dr. Aaron Haas polled young people on the subject of pornography. He asked, "Have you ever read or looked at sexy books or magazines?" A whopping 99 percent of the boys and 91 percent of the girls said yes. Haas found curiosity to be the prime motivation for initially seeking out pornographic material.[1]

It's a fact that most of us have been drawn by curiosity to seek out a pornographic magazine or movie. Just because a person has read a dirty magazine or seen a dirty movie doesn't make him or her a pervert. However, continued and constant obsession with pornographic material can be dangerous. When speaking on the subject of tortures, sex perversions, and murders, former Detroit police inspector Herbert Case said, "There has not been a sex murder in the history of our department in which the killer was not an avid read of lewd magazines."[2] Phoenix, Arizona Police Chief Paul E. Bluebaum said, "Our city has experienced many crimes of sexual deviation such as child molestation and indecent exposure. We find that most of these deviates read obscene material and often exhibit them to the children in an effort to arouse sexual excitement among their victims."[3]

Pornography is a cheapened form of sex. It often treats a human as a sex object. Pornography makes people feel dirty and uneasy about their sexuality. Our sexuality is a gift from God. Sexuality is definitely not the perverted and often quite obscene thing it is portrayed as in so many books and magazines.

When we talk about pornography, we must talk about our minds. I like to use the old phrase "garbage in, garbage out." The principle is simple: If you put garbage into your mind, eventually garbage comes out. The more garbage you put into your mind, the more garbage there is to come out in the form of all kinds of negative behavior. The best way to keep away from a negative thought life and negative behavior is to deprive your mind of garbage. Feed your mind good things, and good things will come out. Feed your mind trash—and guess what comes out? Paul offers some good advice about our thought life: "Finally, brothers, whatever is true, whatever is noble, whatever is right, whatever is pure, whatever is lovely, whatever is admirable—if anything is excellent or praiseworthy—*think* about such things" (Phil. 4:8 NIV, emphasis added).

Some of these bad experiences I've discussed can be avoided; others, unfortunately, cannot be when we are victims of rape or incest. Whatever the specifics of the bad experience you have encountered, get professional help. You don't need to carry around a false sense of guilt or any unhealthy memories of the past. A trained psychologist, a Christian pastor, or a trusted friend can help you, and don't forget that supreme over these helps is God's healing love.

---

### Things to Think About

- What are some things you need to do to protect yourself against rape?
- What things could you do to help a rape victim?
- What new information did you learn about incest from this chapter?
- Why do you think people are so curious about pornography?
- What are specific ways you could apply the "garbage in, garbage out" formula to your Christian growth?

---

# CHAPTER 20

# Questions and Answers

Over the past ten years I've had the privilege of speaking to teenagers and of hearing them talk about their sexuality. Everywhere I go I appreciate their openness, honesty, and sincerity in asking important questions. I have selected some of the questions that have come up most often. My biggest problem in this chapter was keeping it to only fifteen questions!

## 1. Is lust a sin? How can I handle my fantasy life?

Jesus made a strong statement about lust in the Sermon on the Mount. He told his followers, "You have heard that it was said, 'Do not commit adultery.' But I tell you that anyone who looks at a woman lustfully has already committed adultery with her in his heart" (Matt. 5:27-28 NIV). I'm sure that the reason Jesus called lust a sin is that He knew the important part the human mind plays in life. The place to overcome temptation is in your mind. Believe it or not, your mind is your most important sex organ. I'm sure that, at times, everyone has a strong sexual imagination and that, at times, lust barges into everyone's mind. The question is what to do with it when it arrives.

Here are a few brief suggestions for controlling lust and your fantasy life.

- Be assured that you are normal. Nearly everyone you know will have those kinds of thoughts occasionally.
- Don't *feed* your thought life with pornographic magazines, books, films, music, jokes, and so on. I believe that a person can starve his or her fantasy life and cause many of the negative thoughts to go away.
- If you feel completely consumed with lust in your mind, seek the wisdom of a trusted counselor.
- Seek God's help in delivering you from your problem. God is interested in every aspect of your life. Talk to Him about your problems, ask Him for insight and deliverance, and then be open to His answers.
- When you catch your mind beginning to wander, immediately replace those unhealthy thoughts with positive thoughts. Paul's advice in Philippians 4:8 is very good: "Whatever is true, whatever is noble, whatever is right, whatever is pure, whatever is lovely, whatever is admirable—if anything is excellent or praiseworthy—think about such things" (NIV).

2. Is oral sex wrong? What is your opinion of having oral sex instead of intercourse before marriage?

I get asked this sort of question at every seminar I teach on sexuality! My personal opinion is that oral sex is not necessarily wrong in marriage. I believe that if both marriage partners consent and if their sexual exploration is not physically abusive, then it isn't wrong. But when it comes to premarital oral sex, I have a different opinion. I think couples who engage in oral sex are playing with fire. Some couples say it is a form of birth control! I really don't see how a couple can keep from having intercourse if they are experiencing oral sex. It is true that you can't get pregnant from oral sex. The emotional and physical intimacy involved in oral sex, however, is far too similar to intercourse. If your boyfriend or girlfriend gives you the line that oral sex is great and you'll get all the same feelings without intercourse, don't buy that line. Too many people try to make a major distinction between sexual intercourse and oral sex, but the emotions and degree of intimacy are far too similar to clearly separate the two experiences.

**3. Is it possible for sperm to go through my clothing and get inside the vagina?**

The common word for this type of sexual activity is "mutual masturbation." Usually the male is stimulated to ejaculation while rubbing his penis against the female's genitals while one or the other or both still have their clothes on. Many young people practice mutual masturbation as an alternative to the real thing. I think people must be careful to avoid this form of sexual activity. First of all, while it can create a wonderful feeling for the male, the female is usually not as stimulated by this experience. It's very one-sided. Second, mutual masturbation can create negative habits that can carry on into marriage. Premature ejaculation, for instance, is a problem in marriages and is often the result of poor premarital sex habits. Third, mutual masturbation can lead to the real thing. Once you've experienced the "imitation," it's easier to desire the real thing. Fourth, to respond directly to the question, there is a slight chance, depending on the specific garments, that sperm can swim through clothing. But it is not very likely to happen.

**4. Should we get married just because we are having intercourse?**

The answer is no, no, a thousand times no! I've met too many couples (including Christians) in marriage counseling sessions who have told me that the major reason they got married was that they were having premarital sexual intercourse and they felt that it was best to get married instead of continuing to sin. Couples should never get married only to make their sexual intercourse "legal" in God's eyes. That is simply silly, and too many times the marriage ends in disaster. The odds are that if you start a marriage for the wrong reasons, the foundation will crumble and nothing will be left to rebuild the marriage.

Sometimes a guy or girl will try to force the other person into marriage because they are having intercourse. One will try to press guilt on the other. It's true that premarital intercourse is wrong, but two wrongs definitely don't make a right. The best way, then, to tell whether you are getting married for the right reason is to quit having sexual intercourse and see if your desire to marry each other remains as strong as it was.

**5. Are you still a virgin if you had intercourse at age seven but didn't really know what it was? I thought it was a game.**

I believe you are still a virgin. Many young people have innocent sexual encounters when they are really too young to understand much about their sexuality. If this experience constantly bothers you or if the experience was with a relative, you might want to seek counseling to work through any problems the experience has caused in your life. But the majority of people need not feel weird or strange about such an occurrence. Most sexual exploration at a young age is quite innocent.

### 6. How young is too young to get married?

I don't think there is any magical age when marriage becomes right! Since you asked, however, I'll give you a straight answer: Most teenage marriages fail. It may be true that in our parents' day there were more teenage marriages that seemed to work, but the odds are very much against a teenage marriage working out today. Most teenagers do not have the emotional, mental, and spiritual maturity to commit their lives to another person in marriage. They are still growing and changing. One couple I know who was married when they were both seventeen told me that by the time they were twenty-two they had changed so much that they didn't have enough in common to stay married. Yet they were in a heap of trouble because now they had two small children—Tanya, age two, and Kenny, age four—to think about. A divorce would affect all four of them. Now whatever decision they made would involve four people instead of only two.

If you are totally convinced that you must marry as a teenager, make sure that you go through extensive marriage counseling. If you won't do this, I question your maturity. Remember, too, that most teenage marriages fail. I can think of exceptions, but they are not the norm. When I was a teenager, I thought I was mature enough to handle major responsibilities. Now I realize that even though I *thought* I was smart enough to handle something like marriage, I really wasn't. It's a good thing I didn't get married then. I was far too young and immature to be making such a major, lifelong, and life-changing decision.

**7. Is it true that once a guy gets the best of you he's no longer interested?**

I understand your phrase "gets the best of you," but I sure don't like the wording. If a guy is only trying to "get the best of you," then he was never interested in the real you in the first place. But to answer your question, I'm afraid that it is sad but true that some guys do lose respect for and interest in the girl after she has "given in." The girl who "gives in" is taking a major chance that her special friend will lose interest in her. I honestly think that if a girl or guy says, "No, let's wait" and true love is involved, the other person will respect that stand and will be willing to wait. I personally would rather be safe than sorry.

**8. Do guys really want to marry a virgin?**

I think most people would love to marry a virgin. The idea of two people giving one another the special gift of their bodies for the first time in marriage is beautiful and right. All you have to do, however, is look at the statistics to see that perhaps 50 percent of first marriages are not between two virgins. One or both partners have had a previous relationship or they have had premarital intercourse together. Because this is true, it means that as Christians we are called to forgive and to love unconditionally. Just because a person has had sexual intercourse before you met him or her does not necessarily mean that he or she will not be a good marriage partner.

## 9. Is it possible to get the pill without your parents knowing?

At the time of this writing, the answer is yes. According to the "Privacy Act Law," doctors and clinics may issue you the pill without your parents' consent. If you feel you must use a birth control pill, then make sure you talk with a legitimate doctor who can help you make the right decision. I also strongly recommend that you reread the chapter in this book on birth control.

## 10. How often do married people usually have sexual intercourse?

Great question. I always wondered about that when I was in high school, too. It's not as though most of us feel comfortable asking Mom or Dad that question!

Statistics show that some married couples have intercourse once a month and some have intercourse almost every day. Sociologist Ray Short writes that the average number of times per week is three and that the number of minutes per experience, including foreplay and "afterglow," is eight.[1] The average grand total of sexual activity in a given week would be twenty-four minutes! As you can see, if a relationship is primarily based on sex, then there isn't much of a foundation for a positive relationship.

## 11. What is an orgasm?

An orgasm or climax is the peak of excitement in sexual

activity. For a male, the orgasm takes place when the semen is ejaculated from the penis. A female orgasm is a rush of good feelings accompanying a series of vaginal contractions. These contractions may vary in number and in intensity for different people and at different times.

### 12. What is sadism? What is masochism?

Sadism is a mixture of sex and violence. A sadist is a person who gets a kind of sexual pleasure from hurting someone or inflicting pain. Sadism is a sickness, a mental disorder. Keep away from anyone you think might be suffering from this disease. Masochism is another disorder in which a person needs to endure pain and abuse in order to experience sexual pleasure or satisfaction.

### 13. What are the differences between an older guy and a younger teenage girl? Is it safe to date a guy who is seven years older than I am?

The answer, of course, depends on the maturity of the individuals involved. Some seventeen-year-old girls or guys are very mature for their age, and some twenty-four-year-olds still act like thirteen-year-olds. It's my opinion that most of the time a dating relationship between an older guy and a teenage girl doesn't work. I also think there are some important questions to consider in regards to this kind of relationship. Ask yourself, for instance, why would an *adult* seven years older than I am be interested in me? Is there primarily a sexual interest? Is he more serious about the relationship than I am? Will I miss out on some of the fun of high school by dating an adult? What have his past relationships been like?

Even asking this question shows you have some real smarts! I hope you will take a long, slow, rational look at the pros and cons of the relationship and then seek the advice of people you love and trust. Ask a variety of people. Ask people your age. Ask your parents, youth workers, teachers, and anyone else who might have an opinion that you trust. I think my answer would usually be that I'm not sure it is the best thing for you in the long run to date an adult who is seven years your senior. Life is too valuable and short to take many chances when it comes to adult/teenage relationships.

14. Will I suffer any adverse psychological effects if I don't have a boyfriend until college? (It's not my choice! I'd like to have a boyfriend now!)

This is one of the all-time great questions. I appreciate this girl's openness and honesty. I surely do not believe that anyone should or will suffer "adverse psychological effects" because of a lack of dating life in high school. If there were such effects, up to 50 percent of the people in high school would be in big trouble!

I can imagine how hard it must be to really desire to have a boyfriend (or girlfriend) and yet never have that kind of relationship, especially when others are beginning to date. But take heart. Many people never date in high school and others never date in college. I call them "late bloomers." Some of these late bloomers end up having the greatest times in high school and college because they aren't tied down—though they would not have minded a date or two or three or one hundred! It is hard not to be asked to homecoming or the big dance, but unfortunately everyone doesn't get asked.

My advice is don't spend your time waiting for that phone call! Keep busy, keep active—and I'm 100 percent convinced that eventually you'll have a special relationship that will make all the waiting worth it. The worst thing you can do is sulk and retreat from others. This will only cause deep hurt and resentment. I know a number of girls and guys who didn't date in high school and who now have wonderful relationships with those of the opposite sex. I bet you'll have the same thing happen to you.

### 15. Is marijuana dangerous?

I've heard it said for years that marijuana is only a weed, not a drug. It has been said that this weed is basically harmless and that there shouldn't be a big deal about smoking a few joints once in a while. That is simply misinformation, especially in the 1980s. Research tells us that the marijuana used today is ten to twenty times stronger than that available a decade ago.[2]

Researchers today are also concerned that chronic marijuana use might cause permanent damage to the reproductive system as well as various emotional problems. Is marijuana dangerous? For some a joint once in a while may never affect them. For others, that joint could be the beginning of a tragedy. I, for one, am not willing to take the chance.

# CHAPTER 21

# A Frank Discussion With Parents and Youth Workers

A professor at Wheaton College told me recently that when he polled his students about their own sex education he found that only 20 percent had ever had any sex education at home and only 15 percent were taught about sex in their churches. I believe it is very unfortunate that parents and the church have been more or less silent when it comes to sex education. It isn't an easy subject to discuss with our kids, but I believe that our silence is really hurting this generation of young people.

I want to list some alarming statistics that I've taken from a very reputable book entitled *The Private Life of the American Teenager.* The numbers are startling:
- Nearly 6 out of 10 16-18-year-olds have had sexual intercourse
- Nearly 1 out of 3 13-15-year-olds have had sexual intercourse
- The average age for first sexual experience is between 15 and 17
- Nearly 6 out of 10 sexually active teenagers do *not* use birth-control methods, or use them only some of the time
- Nearly *three-quarters* of today's teenagers have *never* discussed birth control with their parents
- Almost *all* teenagers want more information about

intercourse, birth control, and venereal disease (in that order)

- Only 13% of today's teenage girls would marry the father of the baby if they became pregnant. Nearly 3 out of 10 would get an abortion, and the rest would keep the baby or give it up for adoption
- 90% of teenagers surveyed believe in marriage, and 74% say they would live with someone before marriage or instead of marriage.
- Twice as many girls as boys fear that marriage would interfere with their freedom and career plans[1]

With these statistics in mind, how can we as parents and youth workers still remain silent? If you are like me, these statistics frighten you. You and I both know that they are probably true. We are raising a generation of teenagers who are trying to be like sexually active adults but who still make decisions based on teenage emotions. I hope that we adults can be more open and understanding when it comes to helping our young people deal with their sexuality.

We are a curious people. Sex is mysterious and our kids, like ourselves at their age, have a real curiosity and hunger to find out more about their bodies and about sexuality. I think it is a shame that so much of a young person's education must take place in the locker room, through reading *Playboy,* or even in the value-neutral sex education of some public school systems.

## Be Open

I think it's time to open up! It's time to talk about sexuality with our kids. They don't understand it much better than you did at their age, and yet they are probably more sexually involved than any generation before them. After I talked with a group of parents recently about teenage sexuality, though, a parent challenged me by saying, "I'm not sure we should talk to our children about sex. The more information they get, the more curious they become. The more curious they become, the more apt they will be to indulge."

Good thought, but completely wrong. Many young people today do not have the slightest idea how important or sacred their sexuality is. They've bought our culture's lie that "If it feels good, do it." They've never had the privilege of an explanation of what their sexuality is all about. *They need you.* Our young people need you to share with them in an open, honest way about sexuality. They need you to sit with them and really communicate the how and why of their sexuality.

One young person told me recently, "My dad told me not to do it, but he never told me why not to do it and when I did it I was disappointed. I wish he had explained his opinion to me." When it comes to sexuality, I believe firmly that young people who have had an open, honest relationship with their parents and/or youth workers have much healthier attitudes and will find themselves in less trouble in the long run.

## Teach Biblical Sexuality

Biblical sexuality is much more than "God says not to do it!" Biblical sexuality teaches that God created our sexuality—and not only did He create it but He sees it as very good! (See Gen. 1:31.)

We have too many Christian and non-Christian kids today who think that God hates sex. As I've said before, they think He's the great kill-joy in the sky. Often they have these thoughts because no one has ever taken the time to share with them about sex from God's perspective.

We need to communicate to our kids that our bodies and our sexuality are gifts from God (1 Cor. 6:19-20). These gifts should be respected and taken care of. We should teach the biblical view that intercourse before marriage is called sin. Then, keeping in mind the statistics quoted earlier in this chapter, we must make sure our kids learn about grace and forgiveness. I'm afraid most kids are illiterate when it comes to sexuality and the Scripture. You have the rare privilege of giving them the insight that they desperately desire to have.

### Talk About Related Subjects

Believe it or not, your kids want to know your opinion on subjects relating to sexuality. They want to know your thoughts on peer pressure, abortion, dating, unconditional love, the pill, and so on. All of these subjects and others as well are being talked about at school, and both youth workers and parents must deal with these subjects in order to balance out some of the misinformation kids are getting from so-called "experts"—their peers who are making up the story as they go along. I'm afraid that too many times our kids don't listen to us because we always want to give them *the* answer without ever listening to them. Even if the kids are dead wrong, we need to listen to them. When I let kids share their views, they are more open to other views. Sometimes they've never heard other perspectives or even verbalized their own views, and when this happens, the kids often will change their minds!

### Teaching Methods

There are numerous ways to discuss sexuality with

young people. The particular method we use is not as important as the fact that we find time to have open and honest discussions about these important issues. Here are a few ideas to help you develop a more open and honest relationship for talking about sexuality.

Films: Go to a library, a Christian film distributor, or a videotape rental source. Use both Christian and secular films as springboards for discussion.

Books: Read a book together. Good material on sexuality and related subjects is available.

Newspapers: Nearly every day there are articles in the newspaper that can serve as discussion starters.

Classes: Take a human sexuality class together. Many schools offer special courses in sexuality. Take the class with your kids and use the lessons as springboards for continued discussions.

Youth Group Activities: Youth workers can use a number of other valuable learning methods. Case studies can be used very effectively as can questions written out anonymously and answered by the youth workers or parents. Some groups use panel discussions with good results. Many youth workers today will bring in an expert to speak with their groups. You can usually find a youth worker, doctor, nurse, teacher, or psychologist in your area who will do an excellent job of leading a seminar.

The point I'm trying to make in this chapter and in this book is that kids need parents and youth workers to use every method available in teaching about one of the most important subjects to all of us, our sexuality. Keep an open mind, be willing to share your feelings, be open to disagreement, be sensitive to needs—and everyone involved will come out better people. By discussing sexuality with your young people, you may prevent some very negative experiences. You will also be giving the gift of a healthy attitude and godly stewardship of one of God's most special gifts to us, our sexuality.

**Some Helpful Books**
Here are some books which offer additional information and the perspectives of other writers. The list is not exhaustive. I chose these books because they are biblical, easy to read, and still in print at the time of this writing.

Ameiss, Bill and Jane Graves. *Lord of Life, Lord of Me*. St. Louis, Missouri: Concordia Publishing House, 1982.

Kirby, Scott. *Dating: Guidelines from the Bible*. Grand Rapids, Michigan: Baker Book House, 1979.

McDowell, Josh and Paul Lewis. *Givers, Takers and Other Kinds of Lovers*. Wheaton, Illinois: Tyndale House Publishers, 1980.

Olsen, Arvis J. *Sexuality: Guidelines for Teenagers*. Grand Rapids, Michigan: Baker Book House, 1981.

Richards, Larry. *How Far Can I Go?* Grand Rapids, Michigan: Zondervan Publishing House, 1979.

Shedd, Dr. Charles. *The Stork Is Dead*. Waco, Texas: Word Book Publishers, 1980.

Short, Ray E. *Sex, Love, or Infatuation: How Can I Really Know?* Minneapolis: Augsburg Publishing House, 1978.

Souter, John C. *Date*. Wheaton, Illinois: Tyndale House Publishers, 1981.

Stafford, Tim. *A Love Story: Questions and Answers on Sex*. Grand Rapids, Michigan: Zondervan Publishing House, 1977.

White, Mel. *The Other Side of Love: Bible Stories Not for Children*. Old Tappan, New Jersey: Fleming H. Revell Company, 1978.

Wilkerson, David. *This Is Loving?* Ventura, California: Gospel Light, 1972.

# Glossary of Terms

These definitions are provided for your convenience. The words listed are largely restricted to terms used in this book. For help with words not on this list, see a dictionary or some of the books in "Some Helpful Books."

**Abortion:** The premature ending of a pregnancy. There are two types. *Induced abortion* is a medical procedure performed at the request of the woman or her doctor; *spontaneous abortion*, also called "miscarriage," is a natural termination usually due to some problem in the development of the fetus.

**Abstinence:** The voluntary avoidance of something, as in the voluntary avoidance of sexual intercourse.

**Adoption:** The act of taking a person into one's family and raising him or her as one's own child. Unwed mothers sometimes allow their babies to be adopted by others.

**Adultery:** Voluntary sexual intercourse between a married person and a partner who is not the husband or wife.

**Arousal:** Excitement, stimulation.

**Birth control:** *See* Contraception.

**Bisexual:** Pertaining to both sexes; having both male and female sexual organs; sexually attracted to members of both sexes.

**Cervix:** The narrow, lower part of the uterus.

**Climax:** *See* Orgasm.

**Clitoris:** The small, sensitive organ at the upper end of the vulva. It corresponds to the penis.

**Conception:** Impregnation. Penetration of the ovum (female egg cell) by a sperm.

**Condom:** *See* Contraception.

**Contraception:** (Birth control.) The prevention of conception by use of devices or drugs. Commonly used methods are: *Birth control pill*—A drug made of synthetic hormones which prevents ovulation. Available only by prescription; must be used exactly as prescribed. *Condom*—A thin rubber sheath placed over the erect penis before intercourse to prevent sperm from entering the vagina. *Vaginal foam, jelly, suppositories, sponge, etc.*—Non-prescription products, which are applied to the inside of the vagina. Most contain a spermicide—a chemical substance which kills sperm cells. *Diaphragm*—A thin rubber shield which covers the cervix and prevents sperm from entering the uterus. Must be individually fitted by a doctor. *Premature withdrawal*— Withdrawal of the penis from the vagina before orgasm. Largely unreliable because sperm may be released before ejaculation. *Rhythm method*— Abstinence from intercourse during the woman's fertile days as determined by her menstrual cycle.

**Douche:** Cleansing of the vagina with a stream of liquid such as water or other substances.

**Egg:** *See* Ovum.

**Ejaculation:** The emission of semen from the penis.

**Embryo:** An unborn baby from the moment of conception to the beginning of the third month of development. (At this point it begins to be referred to as a fetus.)

**Endocrine:** A gland producing an internal secretion which regulates or controls functions of other parts of the body.

**EPT:** Early Pregnancy Test. Available without a prescription to determine if a girl or woman is pregnant.

**Erection:** The enlargement and hardening of the penis or clitoris as tissues fill with blood.

**Estrogen:** A hormone which promotes the menstrual cycle and affects the development of secondary sexual characteristics in the female (breast development, widened hips, etc.).

**Extramarital:** Outside of marriage. Often used to refer to illicit sexual intercourse—"extramarital affair."

**Fallopian tube:** The tube through which the egg (ovum) passes from the ovary to the uterus.

**Fertilization:** The act of initiating biological reproduction: the penetration of the ovum by a sperm, resulting in conception.

**Fetus:** The unborn child from the third month after conception until birth.

**Fondle:** To stroke or caress with affection.

**Foreplay:** The first stage of a sexual experience, during which partners may kiss, caress, and touch each other in order to achieve full sexual arousal.

**Fornication:** Sexual intercourse between unmarried partners.

**French kiss:** A kiss in which the person's tongue enters the partner's mouth.

**Genital Herpes:** A viral disease that causes blistering of the genital areas; sexually transmitted. (*See* Venereal Disease).

**Genitalia:** (Genitals, genital organs.) The reproductive organs, particularly the external, visible organs such as the clitoris, vulva, and vagina in women and the penis and testicles in men.

**Gonorrhea:** *See* Venereal Disease.

**Guilt:** The fact of being responsible for an offense or wrongdoing; the remorseful awareness of having done wrong. "Real guilt" refers to the fact of having done wrong and to the appropriate awareness of having done so. "False guilt" refers to hanging on to these guilty feelings, being unable to forgive oneself even after the offended party has extended forgiveness.

**Herpes:** *See* Genital Herpes.

**Heterosexual:** A person who is sexually attracted to or

sexually active with persons of the other sex.

**Homosexual:** A person who is sexually attracted to or sexually active with persons of his or her own sex.

**Hormone:** A chemical substance, produced by an endocrine gland, which has a specific effect on the function of other organs in the body.

**Immoral:** Contrary to accepted morality.

**Incest:** Sexual intercourse between close relatives such as father and daughter, mother and son, or brother and sister.

**Infatuation:** A short-lived and superficial attraction to another person.

**Intercourse, sexual:** The act whereby the penis is inserted into the vagina. (Note: the word "intercourse" alone can refer to communication, an exchange of ideas between persons or groups.)

**Masochism:** Cruelty to oneself; receiving sexual pleasure from experiencing pain or harsh domination.

**Masturbation:** Stimulation of one's own sexual organs, often to the point of orgasm.

**Menstruation:** The periodic discharge of blood from the uterus through the vagina.

**Nocturnal Emission:** (Wet dream.) An involuntary occurrence of male erection and ejaculation during sleep.

**Oral sex:** Stimulating the partner's sexual organs with the tongue and/or mouth.

**Orgasm:** The peak of excitement in sexual activity, characterized by a series of muscular contractions.

**Ovaries:** The two female sex glands found on either side of the uterus, in which the ova (egg cells) are formed. They also produce hormones which influence female body characteristics.

**Ovulation:** The release of an ovum (egg) from the ovary to the Fallopian tube.

**Ovum:** (Plural: ova.) The egg, or female reproductive cell, found in the ovary. After penetration by a male sperm, the human egg develops into an embryo and then into a fetus.

**Penis:** The male sex organ through which semen and urine are discharged.

**Pornography:** Literature, films, pictures, or other means of expression which exist solely for the sake of sexual arousal with no concern for personal or moral values.

**Pregnancy:** The period from contraception to birth; the condition of having an embryo or fetus within the body.

**Premarital:** Before marriage.

**Prenatal:** Before birth.

**Procreation:** The act of producing offspring.

**Progesterone:** A hormone which prepares the uterus to receive the fertilized ovum.

**Promiscuous:** Engaging in casual sexual relationships or in sexual intercourse with many persons.

**Prophylactic:** A device or drug used to prevent disease. Common term for the condom.

**Rhythm Method:** *See* Contraception.

**Rape:** Forcible sexual intercourse with an unconsenting partner.

**Sadism:** The need to inflict pain on the partner in order to receive sexual pleasure.

**Semen:** The fluid, containing sperm, which is ejaculated through the penis when the male reaches orgasm.

**Sexual Intercourse:** *See* Intercourse, Sexual.

**Sperm:** The male reproductive cells, produced in the testicles, discharged in the semen through the penis and capable of fertilizing the female egg.

**Spermatic Duct:** (Vas Deferens.) The tube in the male through which sperm passes.

**Spermicide:** A substance that kills sperm.

**Sterilization:** A procedure by which a male or female is rendered unable to produce children; he or she is still able to engage in sexual intercourse. Some common methods are: *Laparoscopy*—An operation in which small incisions are made in the abdomen, allowing the surgeon to cut or cauterize the Fallopian tubes. *Tubal ligation*—An operation in which the surgeon cuts and ties the ends of both Fallopian tubes. *Vasectomy*—An operation in which the male sperm-carrying duct is cut and tied.

**Sublimate:** To modify the natural expression of an impulse, such as sexual desire, in a socially acceptable manner.

**Syphilis:** *See* Venereal Disease.

**Testicles:** The two sex glands in the male which secrete sperm.

**Tubal Ligation:** *See* Sterilization.

**Uterus:** The muscular, pear-shaped female organ in which the fetus develops.

**Vagina:** (Birth canal.) The passage in the female body between the uterus and the vulva. It receives the penis during intercourse and is the canal through which an infant passes at birth.

**Vasectomy:** *See* Sterilization.

**Venereal Disease:** (VD.) Any of a variety of contagious diseases transmitted almost exclusively by sexual intercourse. Some of the most common are genital herpes, gonorrhea, and syphilis.

**Virgin:** A person who has never had sexual intercourse.

**Vulva:** The external genital organs of the female.

**Wet Dream:** *See* Nocturnal Emission.

**Womb:** *See* Uterus.

# Endnotes

**Chapter 1**
None.

**Chapter 2**
**1.** Larry Richards, *How Far Can I Go?* (Grand Rapids, Michigan: Zondervan Publishing House, 1979), p. 96.
**2.** Ibid., p. 43.

**Chapter 3**
**1.** C. S. Lewis, *The Screwtape Letters* (New York: Macmillan Publishing Company, Inc.), p. 83.
**2.** Ray E. Short, *Sex, Love, or Infatuation: How Can I Really Know?* (Minneapolis: Augsburg Publishing House, 1978), p. 83.
**3.** Ibid., p. 83, 88-89.
**4.** Richards, p. 43.

**Chapter 4**
None.

**Chapter 5**
**1.** Bill Ameiss and Jane Graves, *Lord of My Life, Lord of Me* (St. Louis, Missouri: Concordia Publishing House, 1982), p. 75.
**2.** Jane Norman and Myron Harris, M.D., *The Private*

*Life of the American Teenager* (New York: Rawson Wade Publishers, Inc., 1981), p. 54.
3. Ibid., p. 42.

**Chapter 6**
1. Josh McDowell and Paul Lewis, *Givers, Takers and Other Kinds of Lovers* (Wheaton, Illinois: Tyndale House Publishers, 1980), p. 89.

**Chapter 7**
None.

**Chapter 8**
None.

**Chapter 9**
1. Aaron Haas, *Teenage Sexuality: A Survey of Teenage Sexual Behavior* (Los Angeles: Pinnacle Books, 1981), pp. 46-49.
2. Ibid.

**Chapter 10**
1. Scott Kirby, *Dating: Guidelines from the Bible* (Grand Rapids: Baker Book House, 1979), p. 49.
2. Ibid., p. 51.

**Chapter 11**
None.

**Chapter 12**
1. Charlie Shedd, *The Stork Is Dead* (Waco, Texas: Word Book Publishers, 1968), p. 83.

**Chapter 13**
1. James Dobson, *Emotions: Can You Trust Them?* (Ventura, California: Gospel Light, 1980), p. 18.

**2.** Jim Burns, "The Guilt Glob," *Sprint* (Elgin, Illinois: David C. Cook Junior High Curriculum), pp. 1-2.

**Chapter 14**
**1.** Shedd, p. 76.

**Chapter 15**
**1.** Shedd, pp. 61-63.

**Chapter 16**
**1.** David Wilkerson, *This Is Loving?* (Ventura, California: Gospel Light, 1972), p. 40.
**2.** Shedd, p. 72.
**3.** Herbert J. Miles, *Sexual Understanding Before Marriage* (Grand Rapids, Michigan: Zondervan Publishing House, 1975), p. 146.
**4.** Ibid., p. 147.

**Chapter 17**
**1.** Arvis J. Olsen, *Sexuality: Guidelines for Teenagers* (Grand Rapids, Michigan: Baker Book House, 1981), pp. 63-64.

**Chapter 18**
**1.** Tim Stafford, *A Love Story: Questions and Answers on Sex* (Grand Rapids, Michigan: Zondervan Publishing House, 1977), p. 103.

**Chapter 19**
**1.** Haas, p. 182.
**2.** Wilkerson, p. 40.
**3.** Ibid.

**Chapter 20**
**1.** Short, p. 54.
**2.** Rana Rottenberg, "The Care Medic: Answering Ques-

tions About Marijuana Use" (Orange, California: Care
Unit Hospital of Orange, 1980), p. 1.

**Chapter 21**
1. Norman and Harris, p. 42.

# Bibliography

Ameiss, Bill and Jane Graves. *Lord of My Life, Lord of Me*. St. Louis, Missouri: Concordia Publishing House, 1982.

Burns, Jim. "The Guilt Glob," *Sprint*. Elgin, Illinois: David C. Cook Junior High Curriculum, September 1982.

Dobson, James. *Emotions: Can You Trust Them?* Ventura, California: Gospel Light, 1980.

Haas, Aaron. *Teenage Sexuality: A Survey of Teenage Sexual Behavior*. Los Angeles: Pinnacle Books, 1981.

Kirby, Scott. *Dating: Guidelines from the Bible*. Grand Rapids: Baker Book House, 1979.

Lewis, C.S. *The Screwtape Letters*. New York: Macmillan Publishing Company, Inc., 1976.

McDowell, Josh and Paul Lewis. *Givers, Takers and Other Kinds of Lovers*. Wheaton, Illinois: Tyndale House Publishers, 1980.

Miles, Herbert J. *Sexual Understanding Before Marriage.* Grand Rapids, Michigan: Zondervan Publishing House, 1975.

Norman, Jane and Myron Harris, M.D. *The Private Life of the American Teenager.* New York: Rawson Wade Publishers, Inc., 1981.

Olsen, Arvis J. *Sexuality: Guidelines for Teenagers.* Grand Rapids, Michigan: Baker Book House 1981.

Richards, Larry. *How Far Can I Go?* Grand Rapids, Michigan: Zondervan Publishing House, 1979.

Rottenberg, Rana. "The Care Medic: Answering Questions About Marijuana Use." Orange, California: Care Unit Hospital of Orange, 1980.

Shedd, Charlie. *The Stork Is Dead.* Waco, Texas: Word Book Publishers, 1968.

Short, Ray E. *Sex, Love, or Infatuation: How Can I Really Know?* Minneapolis: Augsburg Publishing House, 1978.

Stafford, Tim. *A Love Story: Questions and Answers on Sex.* Grand Rapids, Michigan: Zondervan Publishing House, 1977.

Wilkerson, David. *This Is Loving?* Ventura, California: Gospel Light, 1972.